T0276802

Handbook of Medical Informatics

Handbook of
Medical Informatics

Edited by **Codie Horton**

FOSTER
A C A D E M I C S

New Jersey

Published by Foster Academics,
61 Van Reypen Street,
Jersey City, NJ 07306, USA
www.fosteracademics.com

Handbook of Medical Informatics
Edited by Codie Horton

International Standard Book Number: 978-1-63242-209-5 (Hardback)

Contents

Preface

This book provides state-of-the-art information regarding the field of medical informatics. Information Technology (IT) has revolutionized the daily life of a common man, while medical science has been making rapid progress in understanding disease mechanisms, formulating diagnostic techniques and implementing successful treatment regimen, even for those cases which would have been classified as a poor prognosis a decade earlier. The convergence of information technology and biomedicine has introduced additional dimensions of computerized databases for patient conditions, revolutionizing the way health care and patient information is recorded, processed, interpreted and utilized for improving the quality of life. This book discusses three major elementary issues of medical information acquisition from a patient's and health care professional's point of view, translational approaches from a researcher's viewpoint and finally the application potential as required by the clinicians/physicians. The book encompasses modern issues in Information Technology, Bioinformatics Methods and Clinical Applications. It describes the underlying process of procurement of information in a health system, recent technological developments in biomedicine and the realistic evaluation of medical informatics.

Significant researches are present in this book. Intensive efforts have been employed by authors to make this book an outstanding discourse. This book contains the enlightening chapters which have been written on the basis of significant researches done by the experts.

Finally, I would also like to thank all the members involved in this book for being a team and meeting all the deadlines for the submission of their respective works. I would also like to thank my friends and family for being supportive in my efforts.

Editor

Part 1

Information Technology

Anonymization Approach for Protecting Privacy of Medical Data and Knowledge Management

Asmaa Hatem Rashid and Norizan Binti Mohd Yasin

Department of Information Science, Faculty of Computer Science and IT,
University of Malaya, Kuala Lampur,
Malaysia

1. Introduction

The evolution and development of information and technology have facilitated greater sharing and knowledge management of the collection of electronic information provided by data owners, including governments, corporations, and individuals. Such owners create significant opportunities for knowledge management and information retrieval, thus improving decision-making.Correspondingly; the increase in the use of the Internet and its applications in various aspects of life has led to the need to secure data in the medical and research fields, in government offices, corporations, and individual agencies in various fields. Two questions are addressed in the present study. First, why is there an increasing demand for data sharing and knowledge management? This increasing demand is reflected in the rate of demand for data sharing (Figure 1), which is the base reference data for all users (Gardner and Xiong 2009; El Emam et al. 2011).

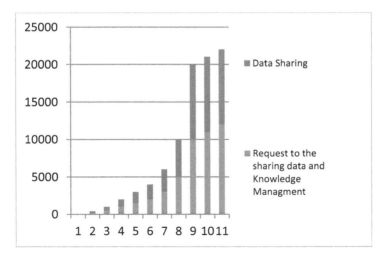

Fig. 1. Require to the Sharing Data and Knowledge Management.

Second, why is there an increase in the control, sharing, and managing of protected or sensitive data for knowledge management? As described in Figure 2, there is a rise in the demand for data sharing, which is the base reference data for all users ((Sweeney 2002)Gardner and Xiong 2009; El Emam, Jonker et al. 2011).

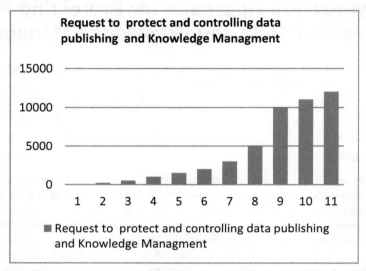

Fig. 2. Require to the protect and controlling data publishing and Knowledge Management.

The above questions imply that both data sharing and knowledge management are indeed on the rise. An increase in the exchange of data leads to the sharing of knowledge and drawing of conclusions based on real data. In turn, data sharing and knowledge management lead to more profit and benefits for service providers and customers. Furthermore, data sharing and knowledge management promote awareness and distribution of knowledge to support decision making in different sectors. Data sharing provides a single source of data to lessen the financial cost in collecting data from research and repeated operations, which require more time and effort. The second question relates to the increase in the control, sharing, and managing of protected or sensitive data and knowledge management. Controlling data exchange and ensuring the security of sensitive data for customers lead to increased trust between the service provider and the customer, promoting their strong relationship in the long run. Information sharing in the medical field supports many decision-making processes.

The strong relationship between patients and the hospital and the link among hospitals lead to better decisions on the management and health of patients. Management of such relationship or Patient Data Management can be assessed using the Customer Relationship Management (CRM) test.

One method that allows health information to be used and declared under existing legal frameworks is de identification. De identification refers to a set of methods that can be applied to data to ensure that the chance of assigning a correct identity to a record in the data is low (El Emam, Jonker et al. 2011).

In performing de-identification, we deduce from the relationship among the size of the data shared, knowledge management, and ways of controlling and sharing data in knowledge management.

A positive or a direct relationship is one that is shared by two parties in which a change in one variable is associated with a change in another variable in the same level. For example, an increase in the volume of data increases mutual knowledge and the control and sharing of data in knowledge management. Figure 3 describes the relationship between the size of data shared and the control and sharing of data in knowledge management (Gardner and Xiong 2009; El Emam, Jonker et al. 2011).

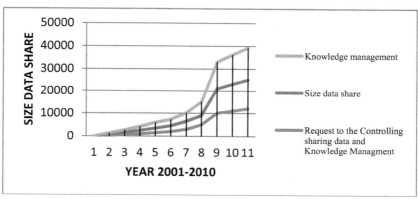

Fig. 3. The Relationship between Data Share Size and Controlling and sharing data of Knowledge Management.

The above motivated us to do work in this area, which will also hopefully encourage research on the control and sharing of data in knowledge management in other fields.

2. Related works

In the past few years, the issue of improving the control and sharing of data in knowledge management has attracted substantial interest among individual users and service providers such as research centers, companies, and governments. This growing interest confirms the importance of the subject and the sensitivity of the work and research involved. Most reviewers and researchers agree on the significant problems present in the control and sharing of data in knowledge management. The problems posed are under more than one research area. These include data confidentiality and privacy protection, with the review of suggested solutions to the problems involving confidential data for cryptographic information and hidden data (Chen and Chu 2008; Kantarcioglu, Jiang et al. 2008), among others. The second area involves data mining and data-mining algorithms to ensure privacy (Bertino, Fovino et al. 2005; Yeh and Hsu 2010), such as generalization and suppression techniques (Hintogdlu and Saygin 2010; Yang and Qiao 2010; Rashid 2010). Other research areas of data management and control of sharing of data ensure integration especially in medical information systems (El Emam, Jonker et al. 2011) and knowledge base systems, which will be the focus of the present study.

In most fields, sharing of data needs the control and management of such data to ensure system integration (Gardner and Xiong 2009), such as patient data, without revealing any sensitive information that can identify a patient. There are several studies that focus on the management of data in medical applications to ensure system integration. However, this can result in information misuse. Nevertheless, there are many algorithms and methods that facilitate management of shared data using techniques such as removing sensitive characters from the information system. Such algorithms are used to prevent unauthorized access to the original data for illicit purposes. In the present research, the main problem is the identification of an algorithm that provides control and management of shared data. Updating current data can be useful for future purposes such as analysis and knowledge management to support decisions in different fields of medical applications; however, the updated data should still represent real cases.

The current study will address this main problem through analyzing and evaluating the following sub problem: There is no model that can identify the number of quasi-identifier characters in such a way that the shared data are managed and a new version of such data is always usable. There is a lack of trust among medical system providers in sharing data and managing knowledge. Aside from the lack of a centralized database to keep the collected data, the problem of case indexing is still left unresolved due to the inability to update data in such a way that it can be used for further analysis and studies. The lack of high-quality updated data and the possibility of errors that adversely affect the results of studies depend on the crucial task of updating the data. As such, the present study attempts to fill in these gaps.

There is a need to build models or design algorithms that manage the sharing of data to avoid misuse. The goal is to bring authenticity to the data system. Guided by recent studies from the years 2005 to 2011 on the control and sharing of data in knowledge management (Fung, Wang et al. 2010), the current work notes that most reviewers and researchers have focused on ensuring the privacy of sensitive data.

In other words, great concern has been directed on the control of data and its sharing to make it available to their owners. Some reviewers and researchers have even suggested the use of covert techniques which isolate data such as encryption technology. Different ways of protecting data have been dealt with in recent research. The methods previously introduced include information on how to spread and use data in research, decision making, scientific analyses, and other purposes (Fung, Wang et al. 2010). First, the concern is how to control data sharing and management and avoid the risk of publishing data that may lead to revealing the real data. Second, there is lack of unity among the collected data, and their sources vary as they are collected from various points such as governments, hospitals, companies, and so on. Third, the data collected may contain errors. How data are processed and formatted before access requires a high level of analysis techniques to extract and determine knowledge and relationships hidden. To identify the relationships among different data and their influence on the results, they must be accurate and correct, as one type of data relies on the results of the analysis.

Examples are the reasons for the spread of a particular disease in a particular area in the medical field, the losses incurred by a company after a change in business strategy, and the low standards of living in a society. The main objective of the present research is to control management and sharing of data in the medical field, which mainly involves "patient data." Our main objective is to propose means to preserve information. The secondary objectives, which relate to the removal of sensitive data, are as follows:

- To evaluate and identify the parameters that negatively affect the management of shared patient data, thus determining the reasons behind the decrease in trust between private and health information communities
- To evaluate and measure the efficiency of k-anonymization and generalization methods in privacy and misuse protection (El Emam, Jonker et al. 2011)
- To build a model that can help prevent shared patient data from being misused
- To test the information metric method using real medical information
- To ensure high-quality information in every stage of the model

Some research questions on the control and sharing of data in knowledge management are as follows: How can data be kept unidentified? How can shared data be managed, ensuring that these benefit the target communities? What indexing methods should be followed to facilitate accurate and fast indexing of a case? How should the effect of perturbation on scientific analysis be measured, and what is an acceptable effect?

3. Information security is not privacy protection

Through this research we would like to clarify the difference between information security and privacy protection, where there is a common area between two subjects where the confidentiality of the data associated with access control and authentication on the received data, which are the traditional areas associated with that in this area recipients of the information has the authority to receive that information.

The problem in this research is more complex and different for the confidentiality of information and very different from the principle of receiving data and how to protect data and which the recipient has the authority receipt.

As the general principle of this research is to release all the data so that the use of data sent or published in scientific fields, but must protect the identities of people who are the landlords of such data or other sensitive properties found in the data). Therefore,(Sweeney 2002).

The aim of this work presented in this research is located outside the traditional work on access and authentication control.

4. Relationship between CRM and control for sharing data

CRM is an integration of people, processes, and technology, which seeks to understand an organization's customers. It is an integrated approach to managing relationships by focusing on customer retention and relationship development.

CRM has been developed from advancements in information technology and organizational changes in customer-centric processes (Chen and Popovich 2003). Figure 4 illustrates the CRM model.

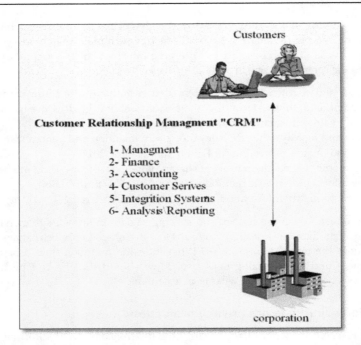

Fig. 4. Customer relationship management (CRM).

Corporations that successfully implement the CRM model gain customer trust and profitability in the long run. However, its successful implementation is unattainable in many organizations mostly because they do not understand that CRM requires organization-wide, cross-functional, and customer-focused business process reengineering (Chen and Popovich 2003).

Usually, CRM is applied in the business field but not in the medical one. The application of the CRM model can result in desirable results through linking the system and the approaches of one hospital with another.

A centralized database is developed, linked with the second database, and then with the third one, thus gathering data from various quarters. Linking of databases allows system integration and facilitates privacy of patient data. Algorithms are used to control sharing of data and knowledge management, as well as maintain privacy of patient data. Using CRM, research in the medical field is simplified by providing one data flow source. CRM encourages scientific research, supports the conclusions gained from the data, and saves patients' time and effort when seeking treatment. The approach also aids in finding the best treatment at the lowest cost and shortest time possible. The technology employing CRM is called Patient Relationship Management (PRM). (Figure 5) describe the Integration Hospital Database System.

Considering the advantages gained by CRM institutions, we therefore recommend the use of PRM. Through PRM, patients establish a connection with the organization (hospital) through an integrated approach of controlling patient data sharing and management. By

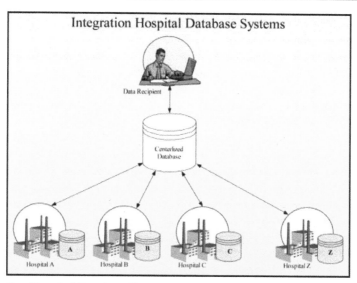

Fig. 5. Integration Hospital Database System.

examining CRM, we learn more about its importance and the advantages and benefits gained by the organizations which use them. We will focus on the processes carried out by the staff in the control of patient data sharing and management.

The following questions arise in the process: How can we control the process of participation and patient data in the medical field? As these data will be collated into a database, this storage combines data from different sources. After the gathering of such data is their organization to form a a knowledge base. We then determine the degree of data privacy involved and the limits to which they can be disclosed so that the identity of the owners of the data can also be protected.

We clarify the process of sending information, for example from a hospital to a central database system, to determine if the divisions have reached integration. To preserve and control the data in this case, we use LeFevre et al.'s (2006) generalization technique. The generalization of the domain values of relational characters to more general values uses the process of distribution of data.

The technique converts the data from private to public while still preserving its usefulness. We delete sensitive information about patients such as their name, identification number, and other details that should be removed, then apply the rules of law agreed upon between the hospital and the patients. Figure 6 provides an example of the generalization technique processing of "patient data" (LeFevre, DeWitt et al. 2005). The general technique includes domain and value generalization hierarchies for zip code (a, b), birth date (c, d), and gender (e, f) (LeFevre, DeWitt et al. 2005).

Using the generalization technique enables us to control the data to be shared and to send it to a central database. After analysis and processing, we provide a knowledge base of real data and results on a scientific basis to provide general information for research and other measures that need the results based on real data.

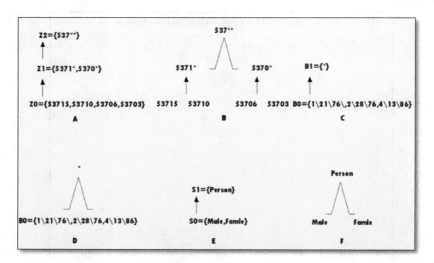

Fig. 6. Domain and value generalization hierarchies for Zip code (a, b), Birth Date (c, d), and Sex (e, f)(LeFevre, DeWitt et al. 2005).

Privacy is addressed by preventing distribution rather than integrating privacy constraints into the data sharing process. Privacy-preserving integration and sharing of research data in health sciences have become decisive in enabling scientific discovery as cited in Sharing Scientific Research Data (Clifton, Kantarcio lu et al. 2004).

5. State-of-the-art privacy preserving

We briefly review the most relevant areas below and discuss how our work levels up with current state-of-the-art systems.

5.1 Privacy preservation in data publication.

The preservation of privacy when publishing data for centralized databases has been examined intensively in recent years. One thread of work aims at devising privacy principles such as k-anonymity and subsequent principles that address problems, which in turn serve as criteria for judging whether a published data set enables privacy protection (Sweeney 2002; Nergiz and Clifton 2007). Another body of work has contributed to the development of an algorithm that transforms a data set to meet one of the privacy principles (dominantly k-anonymity). However, most of these works have focused only on structured data (Li, Li et al. 2007; Xiao and Tao 2007; Gardner and Xiong 2009).

5.2 Medical text de-identification

In the medical informatics community, there have been efforts in deidentifying medical text documents (Sweeney 2002; Zhong, Yang et al. 2005; Gardner and Xiong 2009). Most of them use a two-step approach which extracts the identifying characters first and then removes or masks the attributes for deidentification purposes. Most of them are specialized for specific document types, for example, pathology reports only (Zhong, Yang et al. 2005; Gardner and Xiong 2008). Some systems focus on a subset of Health Insurance Portability and Accountability Act (HIPAA) identifiers, for example, name only (Aramaki, Imai et al. 2006; Gardner and Xiong 2009), whereas others focus on differentiating protected health information (PHI) from non-PHI (Gardner and Xiong 2009). Most importantly, most of these studies rely on simple identifier removal or grouping techniques, and they do not take advantage of recent research developments that guarantee a more formalized notion of privacy while increasing data utility.

5.3 Information extraction

Extracting atomic identifiers and sensitive characters (such as name, address, and disease) from unstructured text such as pathology reports can be seen as an application of the named entity recognition (NER) problem (Neumann 2010). NER systems can be roughly classified into two categories, both of which are applied in medical domains for deidentification. The first uses grammar-based or rule-based techniques (Gardner and Xiong 2008). Unfortunately, such hand-crafted systems may take months of work by experienced domain experts, and the rules will likely change for different data repositories. The second category uses statistical learning approaches such as support vector machine (SVM)-based classification methods. However, an SVM-based method such as that introduced by Sibanda and Unuzer (Sibanda and Uzuner 2006) only performs binary classification of the terms into PHI or non-PHI. It does not also allow statistical deidentification which requires knowledge on different types of identifying characters.

6. Novelty and technical contribution

In the following, we explain the novelty and technical contributions of the survey to data privacy through the control and sharing of data in knowledge management. We focus on six aspects of technical contributions, which we consider to be the most interesting (Xiao 2009).

6.1 Personalized privacy preservation

We examined the work of (Xiao and Tao 2006) on the publication of sensitive data using generalization, the most popular anonymization methodology in the literature. The existing privacy model for generalized tables (that is, noisy microdata obtained through generalization) exerts the same amount of protection on all individuals in the data set without catering to their concrete needs. For example, in a set of medical records, a patient who has contracted flu would receive the same degree of privacy protection as a patient suffering from cancer, despite the willingness of the former to reveal his/her symptoms directly (mainly because flu is a common disease) (Xiao and Tao 2006). Motivated by this, we propose a personalized framework that allows each individual to specify his/ her preferred privacy protection in relation to his/her data. Based on this framework, we devised the first privacy model that considers personalized privacy requests. We also developed an efficient algorithm for computing generalized tables that conform to the model. Through extensive experiments, we show that our solution outperforms other generalization techniques by providing superior privacy while incurring the least possible information loss (Xiao and Tao 2006).

6.2 Republishing dynamic data sets

Data collection is often a continuous process, where tuples are inserted into and deleted from the microdata as time evolves. Therefore, a data publisher may need to republish the microdata at multiple times to reflect the most recent changes. Such republication is not supported by conventional generalization techniques because microdata are assumed to be static (Xiao and Tao 2007). We address this issue by proposing an innovative privacy model called m-invariance which secures the privacy of any individual involved in the republication process, even against a rival who exploits the correlations between multiple releases of the microdata. The model is accompanied by a generalization algorithm whose space and time complexity are independent of the number n of generalized tables that have been released by the publisher. This property of the algorithm is essential in the republication scenario, where n increases monotonically with time (Xiao and Tao 2007).

6.3 Complexity of data anonymization

We have presented the first study on the complexity of producing generalized tables, which conform to ℓ-diversity, the most commonly adopted privacy model. We note that achieving ℓ-diversity with minimum information loss is NP-hard for any ℓ larger than two and any data set that contains at least three distinct sensitive values. Considering this, we developed an $O(\ell.d)$-approximation algorithm, where d is the number of QI characters contained in the microdata (Xiao 2008). Aside from its theoretical guarantee, the proposed algorithm works fairly well in practice and considerably outperforms state-of-the-art techniques in several aspects (Xiao 2008).

6.4 Transparent anonymization

Previous solutions for data publication consider the idea that the rival controls certain prior knowledge about each individual. However, they overlook the possibility that the rival may also know the anonymization algorithm adopted by the data publisher. Thus, an attacker can compromise the privacy protection enforced by the solutions by exploiting various characteristics of the anonymization approach (Xiao 2008). To address this problem, we propose the first analytical model for evaluating the disclosure risks in generalized tables under the assumption that everything involved in the anonymization process, except the data set, is public knowledge. Based on this model, we developed three generalization algorithms to ensure privacy protection, even against a rival who has a thorough understanding of the algorithms. Compared with state-of-the-art generalization techniques, our algorithms not only provide a higher degree of privacy protection but also satisfactory performance in terms of information distortion and overhead estimation (Xiao 2008).

6.5 Anonymization via anatomy

While most previous work adopts generalization to anonymize data, we propose a novel anonymization method anatomy which provides almost the same privacy guarantee as generalization does. However, it significantly outperforms it in terms of the accuracy of data analysis on the distorted microdata (Xiao and Tao 2006). We provide theoretical justifications for the superiority of anatomy over generalization and develop a linear time algorithm for anonymizing data via anatomy. The efficiency of our solution was verified through extensive experiments.

6.6 Dynamic anonymization

We propose dynamic anonymization which produces a tailor-made anonymized version of the data set for each query given by users; the anonymized data increases the accuracy of the query result. Privacy preservation is achieved by ensuring that no private information is revealed despite combining all anonymized data (Xiao 2008). For example, even if the rival obtains every anonymized version of the data set, he/she would not be able to infer the sensitive value of any individual. Through extensive experiments, we show that compared with existing techniques, dynamic anonymization significantly improves the accuracy of queries on the anonymized data (Xiao 2008).

7. Models to control the publication of data

After reviewing the models used in previous research and determining the results of the present study, we make a comparison between the results of the sample and those of different disciplines. Some of the findings were categorized under the confidentiality and privacy of data, whereas others were categorized under the control of post-data.These models are as follows. After searching and accessing a number of studies, we found models used to protect data and those that manage the privacy of data. This step helped us develop and improve the privacy and dissemination of data that can be used in various disciplines while maintaining the same degree of privacy needed (Bugliesi, Preneel et al. 2006; Fung, Wang et al. 2010). the following table describes Models to control publishing of data.

NO.	MODEL NAME
1	k-Anonymity
2	Multi R k-Anonymity
3	ℓ Diversity
4	Confidence Bounding
5	(a; k)-Anonymity
6	(X; Y)-Privacy
7	(k; e)-Anonymity
8	(€;m)-Anonymity
9	Personalized Privacy
10	t-Closeness
11	£, Presence
12	(c; t)-Isolation
13	E-Differential Privacy
14	(d; y)-Privacy
15	Distributional Privacy

Table 1. Models to protect and controlling data publishing (Fung, Wang et al. 2010).

In today's information society, given the unprecedented ease of finding and accessing information, protection of privacy has become a very important concern. In particular, large databases that include sensitive information (e.g., health information) have often been available to public access, frequently with identifiers stripped of in an attempt to protect privacy. However, if such information can be associated with the corresponding people's identifiers, perhaps using other publicly available databases, then privacy can be seriously violated.

For example, (Sweeney 2002)pointed out that one can find out who has what disease using a public database and voter lists. To solve such problems, (Samarati and Sweeney 1998)have proposed a technique called k-anonymization. In this research, we study how to enhance privacy in carrying out the process of k-anonymization.

8. The framework of the proposed model for controlling and managing data sharing

The framework suggested by the present work consists of three stages. As explained in Figure 7, the first stage is when the provider sends data from different databases into an expert database. At this stage, the problem is how to preserve the confidentiality of data sent to the main database. We assume that the connection between the data provider and the centralized database is characterized by trust (Rashid 2010).

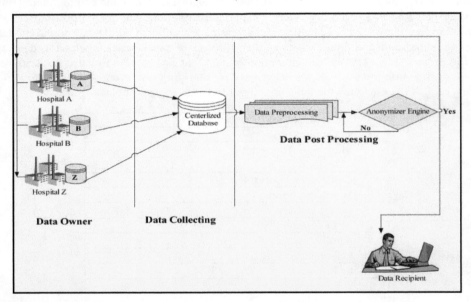

Fig. 7. the Proposed Model to protecting and controlling and manage data sharing.

The second stage is when the expert receives data in the database and recreates (reprocesses) these before sending to the anonymizer engine that applies the k-anonymization and generalization technique. Thus, the second stage is designed for preparing and obtaining data.

The third stage applies data mining algorithms such as analysis, which should identify the hidden relationships among various data and extract results supporting scientific research and decision making. The last stage is the publication of the results on the Web site.

The interface used (published data) and the last version (results) should appear in a simple style to ensure understanding by the recipient (Rashid 2010).

9. Discussion

The purposes of the study on field data anonymization and knowledge management are to allow the release of scientifically useful data in a form that protects the privacy of its subjects and publish knowledge based on real data. Implementing these goals requires more than simply removing personal identifiers from the data because an attacker can still use auxiliary information to infer sensitive individual information.

Additional perturbation is necessary to prevent such inferences, and perturbation of the data in a way that preserves their analytical utility is of significant importance. The great challenge in producing an anonymization scheme is the provision of adequate privacy protection while minimally affecting the analytical utility of the data, which is difficult to doing general and even more difficult to do with high dimensional data.

We previously introduced the observation that anonymity is not required to operate the original data source and proposed that transformation to a prudently chosen source can yield the proper combination of privacy protection, analytical utility, and computational efficiency of anonymization. Studies on data privacy protection have yielded basic criteria with which the degree of privacy required can be measured while maintaining the scientific usefulness of data analysis. The benefits of research and its importance in scientific development and the collection of analytical data based on real medical cases help promote and disseminate knowledge that could assist in the processes of scientific research and raise the level of understanding of the beneficiaries of the research results.

The following questions were raised during the course of our research: Why there is a growing demand for data exchange and knowledge management? How can the demands for controlled data sharing and knowledge management be met? Future research to yield real data can provide answers to these questions and encourage data providers to allow the exchange of personal data for scientific purposes while preserving privacy and sensitive data.

10. Conclusion

This work demonstrates the effort needed to set up a policy framework for the control and sharing of data in knowledge management in the medical field. Data sharing can help guide the nation's adoption of health information technologies and improve the availability of health information and the quality of health care. The proposed control and sharing of data in knowledge management uses the k-anonymization model and generalization technique. The efficiency of these processes has been confirmed through the study and analysis of all processes involved and recent scientific research in the same domain. The control and sharing of data in knowledge management of medical information secure data between health care consumers and providers. The broad use of the proposed system has the potential to improve health care quality and prevent medical errors, thus increasing the efficiency of the care provided and reducing unnecessary health care costs. Moreover, the proposed system would increase administrative efficiency, expand access to affordable care, improve people's health, and provide relevant data to support scientific research.

11. References

Aramaki, E., T. Imai, et al. (2006). *Automatic deidentification by using sentence features and label consistency*.

Fung, B., K. Wang, et al. (2010). "Privacy-preserving data publishing: A survey of recent developments." *ACM Computing Surveys (CSUR)* 42(4): 1-53.

Gardner, J. and L. Xiong (2008). *HIDE: An integrated system for health information de-identification*, IEEE.

Gardner, J. and L. Xiong (2009). "An integrated framework for de-identifying unstructured medical data." *Data & Knowledge Engineering* 68(12): 1441-1451.

LeFevre, K., D. J. DeWitt, et al. (2005). *Incognito: Efficient full-domain k-anonymity*, ACM.

Li, N., T. Li, et al. (2007). *t-closeness: Privacy beyond k-anonymity and l-diversity*, IEEE.

Nergiz, M. E. and C. Clifton (2007). "Thoughts on k-anonymization." *Data & Knowledge Engineering* 63(3): 622-645.

Neumann, R. G. (2010). "Information Extraction." *Architecture* 2: 05.11.

Samarati, P. and L. Sweeney (1998). *Generalizing data to provide anonymity when disclosing information*, ASSOCIATION FOR COMPUTING MACHINERY.

Sibanda, T. and O. Uzuner (2006). "Role of Local Context in De-identification of Ungrammatical, Fragmented Text." *North American Chapter of Association for Computational Linguistics/Human Language Technology (NAACL-HLT)*.

Sweeney, L. (2002). "k-anonymity: A model for protecting privacy." *International Journal of Uncertainty Fuzziness and Knowledge Based Systems* 10(5): 557-570.

Xiao, X. (2008). "Privacy Preserving Data Publishing: A Research Summary."

Xiao, X. (2009). "Privacy Preserving Data Publishing: A Research Summary."

Xiao, X. and Y. Tao (2006). *Personalized privacy preservation*, ACM.

Xiao, X. and Y. Tao (2007). *M-invariance: towards privacy preserving re-publication of dynamic datasets*, ACM.

Zhong, S., Z. Yang, et al. (2005). *Privacy-enhancing k-anonymization of customer data*, ACM.

2

Innovative Integration of Information Systems for Managing a National Access to Surgery

Luís Velez Lapão
Instituto de Higiene e Medicina Tropical, Universidade Nova de Lisboa,
CINTESIS: Center for Research in Health Technologies and Information Systems,
Universidade do Porto,
Portugal

1. Introduction

Leverage technology in improving access to surgery

National Health Systems are facing very difficult times. In most OECD countries, there are evident trends such as the shortage of human resources (HR), HR are becoming too expensive to handle, new therapies that are very expensive and patients that are becoming older and with increasing co-morbidities, and complementary exams that are also very expensive (Gauld & Derret, 2000). It is difficult do cope with the patients demand, to do so managing tools are required. The Portuguese National Health System (NHS) services aims at serving all citizens. The primary-care services cover the entire country and are responsible for referring to hospitals. The larger demand and the limitations of supplying health services lead to the existence of waiting lists (WL). In the case of surgery it leads to waiting lists for surgery (WLS). The spread of healthcare units and of patient demand across the country leads to inefficiency (Porter and Teisberg, 2007). In this regard, the need for information systems (IS) to address the exchange of information between different health institutions is critical (Lapão, 2007).

Today, most of the inefficiency problems relate to the lack of coordination between systems due to the use of different architectures and standards (Lenz and Kuhn, 2002). The National Health Systems Administration (ACSS) is both responsible for addressing the "National Health Information Systems Infrastructure" and developing the "Surgery Access National Program". ACSS started to implement the SIGIC (Integrated System of Management of the Waiting List for Surgery) program in 2005, following a less integrated equivalent program named PECLEC that had started years before. By "access to healthcare" is meant the possibility that individuals have to get proper healthcare treatment according to their needs in order to have real healthcare gains (EOHSP, 2009). In Portugal, access to healthcare services is a constitutional right. Proper care treatment is understood as a combination of factors: the opportunity (on-time treatment), the gains in health (effectiveness), the adequate costs (efficiency), and the value perceived by the patient. The need for regulation elapses from the fact that healthcare services are a scarce and valuable resource. SNS needs to deal with limited resources to serve our 10 million inhabitants: the numbers of primary care health centers in the public healthcare system in Portugal. The numbers of hospital beds in the public healthcare system (regarding North, Centre, Lisbon, Alentejo and Algarve Regions) is limited to 18.553 (MS). The numbers of National Reference System for Continued Integrated Care (RNCCI) beds (North, Centre, Lisbon, Alentejo and Algarve Regions) are limited to 2851 in total. All of these resources (primary care referencing, hospital and tertiary beds availability, surgery scheduling) need proper and timely management (Lapão & Dussault, 2011).

Therefore it became clear that an information system was a necessity. An IS that would integrate the available information about the demand and supply, and at the same time would present an estimate of the patients and the waiting time on the WLS, accessible to professionals and patients. In 2004, SIGIC was defined legally to be a structure of the Ministry of Health to manage and improve the "access to surgery". SIGIC was established to assure the treatment by services in the following terms (PRLD, 2007):

- High standards of technical quality for the healthcare services (quality);
- Maximum allowed waiting time by medical priority and pathology (standards);
- Universal schedule rules safeguarding medical priority and waiting time (equity);
- Guarantees of alternative choice if waiting time is 75% of the maximum waiting time established (process);
- Transparency and guarantee of information quality (transparency).

This chapter contributes to the understanding of the role of information systems integration in supporting the development of a nation-wide access to surgery system. The information system allows for significant improvements in the management with clear impact for patients.

This chapter will start covering the definition of the problem of the management of a nation-wide waiting list system, followed by the definition of an information strategy, and the development of the system to accomplish that aim. At the end the results of the first 5 years of this program will be presented and discussed.

2. The problem of managing nation-wide waiting list for surgery

2.1 The patient path and waiting lists for surgery

Waiting lists (WL) are the register of patients who have been clinically assessed as needing elective surgery in a hospital. It could include patients both with and without a scheduled date of admission to hospital (GoSA, 2006). Since there is an instable equilibrium between demand and services supply, WL is an important and useful management instrument to help prioritize the use of resources in the health system. More important is the rationale behind determination of the waiting time of the patients expecting (queuing for) elective surgery, with the identified problems of clinical urgency and universal access. Furthermore, although the waiting experience was described as stressful and anxiety provoking, for a significant numbers of patients the experience of waiting was not uniformly negative (Carr et al., 2009).

In many western societies the universal access to health services is a constitutional right (EOHSP, 2009). This is an increasingly difficult challenge. Health managers have to use WL management tools aiming at providing the support for proper hospital production planning (Valente & Testi, 2009; van Ackere & Smith, 1999). The adequate use of WL could provide a balanced (and fair) prioritization of patient needs and at the same time provide some pressure over the health system to improve its organization and processes towards a better response, to better reply to the patient demand (Sibbald et al., 2009). To better understand the role of processes and information flow it is important to be aware of the patient path in the system. Figure 1. shows the path of the patient and the time waiting from booking to surgery.

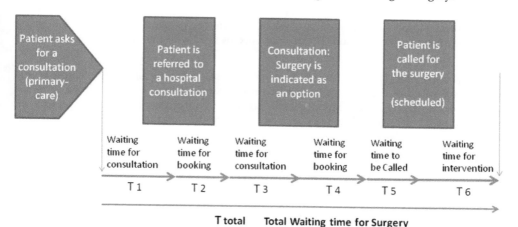

Fig. 1. The patient path in the system.

We have split the total flow in six stages with the corresponding time (Ti). The first stage starts when the patient initiates the consultation booking process in the eAgenda system (available in the Internet), where he/she can pick-up one available spot within the next days. T_1 is the time the patient will wait until the consultation in the health centre. The second stage starts when the family physician considers that the patient probably requires a surgery and decides to refer the patient for a hospital consultation. T_2 is the time the patients need to wait before the hospital consultation is effectively booked. When the booking is completed, patient will have to wait until the hospital consultation (T_3). The third stage starts with the indication for surgery by the hospital surgeon, after which the patient will have to wait until the surgery is booked (T_4). After that patient will have to wait to be called for the procedure (T_5), then the surgery is scheduled. After the surgery is been scheduled the patient will have to wait until the actual day of the procedure (T_6).

The total waiting time for surgery T_{total} is the linear summation of the six partial times: T_{total} = $T_1 + T_2 + T_3 + T_4 + T_5 + T_6$. The management problem here emerges from the fact that we do not have enough information about any of these waiting times. Recently, the introduction of eAgenda, Alert (used for supporting the referring process) and other systems created the opportunity for getting closer to the situation, nevertheless the databases are not prepared to be used for management analysis. These information systems were built for the unique purposed of exchanging information rather than allowing for tactical and strategic analysis.

2.2 Wanting list theory

A "waiting list" is the collection of random arrivals of patients (demanding for a surgery) and the necessity of allocating the right resources to avoid waste and inefficiencies (intervention capacity not used) (GoSA, 2003). This organizational capacity must be managed in order to properly satisfy the needs of patients without exceeding the recommended or acceptable waiting time (taking much time than clinical recommended or acceptable). We should use the total waiting time (T_{total}) as one suitable indicator of performance. This indicator is clearer than the total number of inscribed patients because it really tells the impact on patient's life, while the number of patients in the WLS is just a number expressing the demand. It does not specify how well the systems respond to the demand.

A long waiting time (T_{total}), if longer than recommended for the pathology, could be the result of an excess of demand and a lack of resources to properly respond. In the case of a weak response the Health authorities are require to intervene to tackle the problem. Nevertheless, to manage an intervention is necessary to develop mechanisms for controlling both the demand and the supply. On the one side, the demand depends from non controllable factors such as population health status, available resources and the clinical practice. On the other side, controlling the supply by hospital services could mean to improve capacity, by either using more resources or by increasing efficiency. If necessary, hospital managers could also increase capacity temporarily to tackle a punctual problem of excess of the demand.

As a theory, Iversen (1993) proposes the need to consider that the no-cooperative character of resource allocation in a national health service could contribute to excessive waiting lists. The theory of hospital waiting lists is derived from this concept. The existence of waiting lists implies the loss of efficiency: the hospital's resources are drawn away from medical work. Although there is scope for Pareto improvements, the structure of budget allocation obeys other criteria and may prevent these improvements from being achieved. The health organization may need to be re-organized. Therefore, the conceptualization of a nation-wide system for managing the access to surgery will need rethinking (and the Surgical Departments should also review their processes).

Health services could use waiting lists in general for different purposes, being one of the most relevant the waiting list for (elective) surgery (WLS). An elective surgery is a surgery that, once established as an indication, can await over 24h before being performed, note that it does it cover medical treatments other than specific stabilizing drugs in preparation for surgery. Opposed to this definition is emergency surgery or treatment, which needs performing within less than 24h. WLS should encompass specific instruments to help hospital's managers' process the patients enrolled, their established surgical indication and its priority time frame.

With increasing life expectancy and of co-morbidities, the demand for new hospital specialist consultations is huge. This demand could arrive to the hospital through two different pathways: either by referral from primary health care or by direct entrance in the emergency. However, in the case of elective surgery, the patients usually enter from primary care referral. The demand for hospital specialty consultations increases from primary-care referral, leading to an increase in hospital consultations, some of them leading to the WLS, others to other types of treatment. The later produce an increase in the waiting time for booking and consultation (T2 and T3). If the number of surgeries performed does not cope with the increasing demand, it leads to a further increment in the number of patients registered in the WLS. Before the introduction of mechanisms for managing waiting lists, often cases would go to media because a patient had died before proper treatment had been delivered, or because other patient had stayed in the list for months, much longer than guidelines recommended. These situations are unacceptable by public opinion and pressure built-up for governments to introduce sophisticated mechanisms to support a fair approach to improve access to surgery. These mechanisms are also important to assure transparency in processes regarding selection and scheduling patients to surgery. Furthermore, by allowing for complete registration of the process, this new system will render accountable those responsible in cases of longer than expected waiting time.

One of the purposes of the system is to integrate data from all patient surgeries registrations, independently of other requirements like the need for staying in the hospital as inpatients, type of anesthesia to be used, or where the surgery will be performed (in a NHS hospital or on a private or social institution). In order to improve workflow the patients have to sign the express his/her consent before registration in the WLS. Signed consent is also needed for legal purposes. Hence, a system for managing the access to surgery is supposed to regulate all the programmed surgery production and incorporate the whole set of stages in patient management.

2.3 The negative health effects of a long permanence in the waiting list for surgery

The existence of a significant number of patients waiting for treatment that exceed the clinical acceptable times has ominous consequences not only for the individuals (increasing suffering, reduce treatment success, more complex treatments) but also for the society (more expensive use of resources, higher absenteeism, etc), which forced the government to take political measures such as the creation of an upgraded program.

In the recent past, the access to healthcare was carried through in a non-regulated manner and the integration of the different levels of treatment was inexistent. The citizen did not have the opportunity to be aware of the process. The system evolved, with the expansion of new regulation units guided towards efficiency of the system centered in the patient. Health-care referencing nets were defined and consolidated and the participation of the patient was strengthened during the development of the processes (Jeston and Nelis, 2006). It is put together as a comprehensive system that integrates the diverse levels of healthcare.

The regulation should be centered on patient gains in health. As the Portuguese National Health service is driven by the "Primary-care", closer to patients, from which MCDT (Exams, Complementary Means of Diagnosis and Treatment) are prescribed and hospital-care is referenced. SIGIC personnel works the data from surgical services, medical services, and other MCDT in order to manage the "surgery access" (with SIGA: the Integrated System of Management of the Access) and related it with Continued care and, Patient needs.

2.4 Problems managing waiting lists

Prioritization of waiting lists for elective surgery represent a major issue in public systems in view of the fact that patients often suffer from consequences of long waiting times (Valente et al., 2009). The most significant problem whilst managing waiting lists is to access all the important information to accelerate the decision process (take faster decisions) (Dexter et al., 2000). But, when there are plentiful resources available often the easy solution to "through money" into the problem. This was the case for the first years of addressing the waiting list for surgery. In Portugal, since 1995 four interventions have been developed to tackle WLS. First, PERLE (Waiting Lists Solution Specific Program) run from 1995 to 1998. Second, in 1999, it was launch the PPA (Access Promotion Program) with small improvements. Third, in 2001, a more sophisticated PECLEC (Surgery Waiting Lists Reduction Special Program), with specific reduction goals was initiated. These first three experiments programs would lead to the fourth intervention with SIGIC (that will be analyzed in the following pages).

3. Evidence from what others have done

Siciliani & Hurst (2004) found that waiting times may be reduced by acting on the supply of or on the demand for surgery (or both). Van Ackere & Smith (1999) proposed a macro model for developing a National waiting lists management system. They mentioned that waiting lists for surgery have been endemic to the UK National Health Service since its inception in 1948. The use of waiting lists reveals a management concern to serve the patients. The lists emerge as a result of interaction between supply factors (the provision of resources and the efficiency of their use) and demand factors (arising from a complex conjunction of the perceptions and preferences of patients and physicians). The adoption of a macro model takes an economic perspective and assumes that the waiting time for surgery, as perceived by patients, physicians and managers, is a central influence on the quantity of elective surgery demanded and supplied. From their study, van Ackere & Smith (1999) further alert, by exploring a number of future scenarios, for the fact that the NHS will eventually cease to be a universal service if resources fail to keep pace with increasing demand.

VanBerkel & Blake (2007) performed a comprehensive simulation for waiting time reduction and capacity planning applied in general surgery, using operational research techniques. They have studied the consequences of redistributing beds between sites, and achieving standard patient lengths of stay, while comparing them to current and additional resource options. This simulation exercise proved that there were multiple independent and combined options for stabilizing and decreasing the waiting for elective procedures.

Valente et al. (2009) developed a model to prioritize access to elective surgery on the basis of clinical urgency and waiting time. They mentioned that administrative and standardized data on waiting lists are generally lacking in Italy, even since 2002 an implicit Urgency-Related Groups (URGs) associated with Maximum Time Before Treatment (MTBT) was defined. The Surgical Waiting List Info System (SWALIS) project was created in 2001, with the aim of experimenting solutions for managing elective surgery waiting lists. First, only ten surgical units in the largest hospital of the Liguria Region were involved in the design of a pre-admission process model embedded in web-based software. This SWALIS system allowed pre-admissions based on several steps: 1) urgency assessment into URGs; 2) correspondent assignment of a pre-set MTBT; 3) real time prioritization of every referral on the list, according to urgency and waiting time. Next, they selected a single surgery unit to perform a prospective study, from March 2004 to March 2007 (1809 ordinary and 597 day cases). The study lead to the change in the SWALIS model: waiting lists were monitored and analyzed, measuring a significant impact of the model by a set of performance indexes (average waiting time, length of the waiting list). The SWALIS pre-admission model was used for all registrations in the test period, fully covering the case mix of the patients referred to surgery. The software produced real time data and advanced parameters, providing patients and users useful tools to manage waiting lists and to schedule hospital admissions with ease and efficiency. Positive changes were observed, meaning that more patients were treated within their MTBT. The SWALIS model managed to provide useful data to monitor waiting lists and it also allowed a standardized prioritization of patients, an enhancing transparency, more efficiency and equity.

Kim, S.C. & Horowitz, I. (2002) took advantage of an advance-scheduling property for elective surgeries by exploring whether the use of a daily quota system with a 1-week or 2-week scheduling window would improve the performance of a typical intensive care unit (ICU) that serves patients coming from a number of different sources within the hospital. They have shown that formally linking the scheduling of elective surgeries (as one controllable upstream process) through a quota system, to the downstream ICU admission process, can have beneficial effects throughout the hospital. This shows that management tools like combining a quota system with scheduling improves efficiency.

Cromwell et al. (2002) assessed six web-based waiting time information services, with a cross-sectional survey of government websites in countries with publicly funded hospitals, to identify how they aimed to meet the information needs of patients and general practitioners, and to evaluate how well waiting time information was presented. The services presented information to help both GPs and patients deciding where to look for a surgery by comparing hospitals statistics. The websites overall advice was poor: the websites did not state whether the statistics predicted expected waiting times, and only one stated that the statistics were only intended as a guide. Statistics were based on different types of data, and derived at different levels of aggregation, raising questions of accuracy. Most sites explained waiting list terms, but provided inadequate advice on the uncertainty associated with making statistical inferences. Cromwell et al. (2002) further suggests that users should access web-based waiting time information services cautiously because of a lack of guidance on how to appropriately interpret the presented information.

Several National Health administrations have addressed the use of information systems to deal with the integration of data but success is still very limited. Most OECD countries use information systems only to monitor the system, whereas health services are obliged to submit regular reports to authorities (OECD, 2003; GoSA, 2006; Kuhn et al, 2007). There is a sense that we are still learning and searching for better solutions to improve the management of access to surgery.

4. Methods: SIGIC and SIGA framework

4.1 SIGIC framework

The need for regulation at the Portuguese National Health System elapses from the fact that healthcare services are a scarce and valuable resource. In this context, SIGIC (Waiting List for Surgery's Integrated Management System) was created to manage the "access to surgery", intending to assure the treatment by services in terms of quality, standards, equity, process and transparency.

SIGIC was established (in April 2004) as an integrated system to manage patients waiting for elective surgery (MS, 2004). The main purpose was to overcome specific fragilities of the NHS and to make it more universal by allowing a global management of the system. By considering both the demand and supply together it would be possible to improve management and to optimize the resources. Covering a substantial part of the supply surgery resources of the NHS it would be possible to allow for a better response to prioritization. This effort was developed by a team who looked at other similar international systems for benchmarking (it included Spain, Denmark, United Kingdom, Canada, Australia and New Zeeland). This research concluded that more than 50% of the OECD countries were focusing their attention on "waiting time for elective surgery". The SIGIG task-force initiated its activities with a comprehensive comparison of international examples. This benchmark exercise was critical to guarantee the best solution would be used to deal with the problem of waiting list for surgery, besides the difficulty of reaching information and of difference and non-homogeneity of concepts used by different systems (Banta & Wija, 2000). There are countries where the struggle for waiting list for surgery is considered a priority in health policy. Comparing Portugal with Spain and United Kingdom there is a clear disadvantage for Portugal both in terms of waiting list and waiting time (TDC, 2007).

The main idea is to centralize the management of the surgical resources offering/enabling the flexibility and the usage of the available resources (specialists, beds, Surgery rooms) leveraging both the public and private hospitals. On the side of demand, it is possible to establish priorities linked with pathologies and their prognosis, creating rules (guidelines) to support the waiting list of surgery management, allowing both the access to public and to private hospitals, if the public ones did not timely respond (MS, 2005).

This sort of strategy is based on the following assumptions (with impact on the IS strategy to be developed):

-   WLS centralized management to allow the optimization of the available resources;
-   Clearly defining institutional aims, regarding maximum waiting time (global and with pathology) and assuring the access to surgery within those maximum waiting time;
-   Promoting alternative methods for performing ambulatory surgeries;
-   Developing incentives and payment models related with surgery production;
-   Promoting a diversification of therapeutic options for patients: from private to social institutions enabling the fulfillment of the clinical goals;
-   Increasing the hospital commitment for releasing the waiting list for surgery certificate (WLS), accepting to solve the patient clinical situation within the time frame corresponding to 75% of the WLS maximum time;
-   Standardizing the WLS management processes to assure both transparency and fairness; and promoting the participation from patients (recognizing both rights and duties) and formalizing with signature the acceptance in being registered on the WLS;
-   Strong promotion of WLS related information to patients, hospital physicians and managers, and to society in general, based on the actual clinical information and transparency.

To mitigate the implementations and deployment risk (Haugen & Woodside, 2010) it was decided to start the system as pilot covering only a limited region in the south of Portugal

(Algarve e Alentejo). First all the available WLS in that region were collected and analyzed and the system was implemented right away. During that time the data from the hospitals of the remaining of the country started being collected as well. This process of collecting data from the system enables the definition of the SIGIC model (MS, 2005).

SIGIC goals are to reduce waiting time for surgery (improve the service), to apply identical standards to all patients (equity in access), to profit from good use of resources (Increase the efficiency) and, to create a national structure of homogeneous information based in a system of data collection (a database) that elapses from the production process (knowledge and transparency). The chosen strategy was the "survey of information systems and technology in Demand / Supply / Resources", the "institutionalization and monitoring of procedural standards for management of the Waiting List for Surgery (WLS)", to provide "evaluation by results" and, to regard the "Correction of deviations to the standard".

4.2 SIGA framework

To fulfill SIGIC's objectives (defined by law) it was created a management model and an information system (IS) to support it. SIGA is the integrated system of management of the access (includes the information model, regulation model, financial model, incentives and penalties). There are four main issues to be accomplished by SIGA: create knowledge, establish the equilibrium between demand and supply, guarantee the equity in access, improve the quality/efficiency, and tackle sustainability. Therefore, the SIGA mission is to serve adequately the citizen's needs of surgical treatment. Presently 66 public hospitals (all with sustainable surgery activity) and 54 private hospitals (with convention with SIGIC) had joined the SIGIC network (now with 3,012 certified users). The SIGA is based on a centralized architecture and has adopted the following principles:

Means to achieve the goals: After setting the goals and defining the targets, the necessary instruments were built in order to pursue them. The main targets identified were: increasing supply of "surgeries", improving the management of WLS (i.e. creating the conditions to improve the use of operating rooms and surgical teams), supply and demand regulation, process improvement, assess the quality of services provided, guarantee of the access for all citizens and, improving the quality of information.

Processes Effort: Right from the beginning of the effort, a strong drive to properly define the right workflow processes was established, by involving all actors within the system. The result was the definition of: "The circuit of the patient in WLS and in hospital transfers" (Figure 2).

The "hospital of origin" of the patient (HO, the hospital where the patient had the first consultation) classifies the patients according to their priority and tries to schedule a surgery for them on time. But, the shortest defined time limit is 15 days for the HO's surgery department to reply to all cases: The HO must then clarify and declare any lack of capacity for coping with the high priority patients in the list. Therefore, it was further defined a time limit of one month for the HO to perform the surgery. Otherwise, if HO cannot schedule the surgery, the patient must be transferred to another hospital within the network (and accepted by the patient): Then, within 1 to 6.75 months, depending on the priority level assigned, the patient should be sent to another hospital.

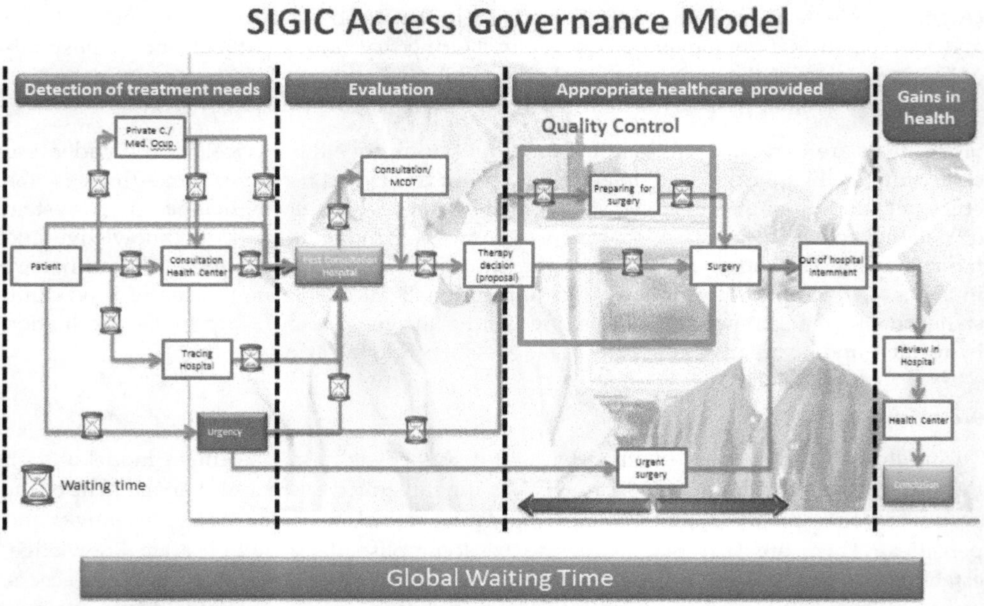

SIGIC Access Governance Model

Fig. 2. SIGIC Access Governance model.

This destination hospital could be a private hospital on the condition of having a convention agreement with SNS/SIGIC. The maximum waiting time allowed was defined as 9 months (always adjusted to pathology). The circuit of each patient is always monitored in order to guarantee that the maximum waiting time is never reached. Once such system is created one should always consider that an increase on apparent demand would be expected. The use of an information system made possible to include all the patients and register them providing a the real perspective of the WL, the patients not previously known, because they were registered in different systems, were tracked and added as well.

In summary, the SIGIC aims at optimizing the demand-supply imbalance by allocating higher priority surgeries to available surgery spots in order to minimize the waiting time for surgery and to address priority surgeries within the clinical expected time.

5. Information systems strategy: From SIGIC to SIGLIC

Once implemented the SIGIC, it was necessary to create an information system for supporting the whole system, allowing for organizing all the data related with surgeries and at the same time to following-up the different stages. It also was necessary to make information available to all partners. It was subsequently decided to develop an information system enabling the storing and the exchanging of all relevant data. This system, designated as SIGLIC (Patient Waiting List Support Information System), is thought to play an important role in coordinating the referring and management processes, with automatism for all standard steps and allowing for transparency and easiness (MS, 2005). SIGLIC is an information system to support SIGA in improving the access to surgery (MS, 2005). The relevance of SIGLIC is that it allows for the complete integration of all SIGIC data and from all set of hospitals. Furthermore, this integration assures the synchronism of data and the interaction of all involved parts.

5.1 Developing an information system strategy

From the perspective of information systems strategy, one could perceive strategy translated as a set of action plus regular improving meetings (Kuperman, 2000). In this sense, the SICLIC is a management decision-making and scheduling information system that was created to support the access to surgery and its clinical and management implications. It was designed to be improved in every cycle of analysis. To develop an information systems strategy a set of main initiatives were identified to be addressed: the design of a clinical and administrative data repository, discovery of inpatient process support, electronic medical records, a web-based portal strategy, selection of referral applications, management of knowledge resources, patient information and participation, confidentiality, and clinical decision support systems.

The SIGLIC is supposed to integrate the data from all hospitals with surgery services, where it picks the data to find optimal solutions for each patient. It should allow for real time exchange of information to drive SIGIC's decision-making processes. SIGIC's goals are to reduce waiting time for surgery, to apply identical standards to all patients, to profit from good use of resources and, to create a national structure of homogeneous information based in a system of data collection. It is important to clearly define who produces and signees for the information, the minimal data set and all the information to be recorded should be included in the workflow (Grilo et al, 2009).

The SIGLIC systems require access to the other hospital and primary care information systems. However this is not a straightforward assignment. The maturity of hospital information systems is still low (Lapão, 2007) and integration barriers is a well-known global problem (Kuhn et al., 2007). The debate over the introduction of Information Systems in healthcare in Portugal at the beginning of the XXI century follows the growing concern that the costs of healthcare are increasing too fast and have already surpassed the acceptable level to society. The pressure for government budget contention from EU is the strongest factor. It all began in the 1990s with major shifts happening from administrative health information systems (HIS) to systems that started to be used by physicians, nurses, and other healthcare providers as part of the delivering process (MS, 1999). But there are also medical reasons to look for the development of an integrated HIS. Western countries, more sensitive to this issue, are witnessing a movement towards the integration of information systems in Hospitals (or preferably integrating the entire healthcare network). In the United States this has been mainly driven by HIPAA, an information privacy and security standard promoted by the US Government, although management reasons are the most relevant due to the opportunity to reduce costs out of inefficiencies (Glaser & Salzberg, 2011). Even in well-advanced countries like The Netherlands (Hasselbring et al., 2000), and the U.K. (McKee & Healy, 2002), there was a perceived lack in actual integration of information systems working as the best practice examples to be followed. There are two fundamental objectives to tackle health information system. First, only recently the management Boards became aware of the hospital management ineffectiveness because they did not have the opportunity to look for proper indicators before (Smaltz et al., 2005; Lapão, 2007; Lapão et al, 2009). The motivation for investing in these systems is now clearly economic and strategic. Physicians and nurses have been encouraged to help the hospital to manage the allocation of resources by a proper cost-benefit analysis of problems. Second, it is also important to acknowledge that Health information systems (HIS) are still quite a complex structure (Winter et al., 2001) that comprehends vast information technologies, several application systems and information management.

A strategic roadmap for SIGLIC Strategy aimed at two objectives: A detailed analysis of the initial WLS situation and the definition of a HIS strategy roadmap, representing an organizational change of hospital surgery-related services that should put the patient and their needs in the centre of the process as well the conditions of healthcare professionals (following the defined business strategy) (MS, 2005). The process started with the SIGIC's mission and objectives definition, both as short and medium term goals. Hence, the board defined that "*The SIGIC's mission is to provide a centralized access to surgery management service, enabling the flexibility and the usage of the available resources (specialists, beds, surgery room) leveraging both the public and private hospitals to globally reduce the waiting list for surgery*"(MS, 2005). Secondly, it is necessary to complete a full-scale characterisation of the surgery-related hospitals information systems that helps to understand the dimension of the task required to reach the goal. Thirdly, regarding the objectives defined for the implementation it is required to address the SIGLIC's strategic alternatives for the integration of the information system considering the SIGIC's specifics. The alternatives were: a) Implement a holistic Solution bought from a HIS supplier; b) Adopt a phased implementation after proper prioritisation; c) Focused only on the most urgent systems; d) Develop internally a system solution that covers all sub-systems requirements.

A very important aspect is how deeply involved in the process the solution provider is and how its leadership is developed throughout the whole process (Smaltz et al., 2005). The providers should be regarded as partners, meaning that the provider should be involved in the process right from the beginning and be co-responsible for the outputs. Mostly because the HIS implementation is part of a crusade to promote the utilisation of the HL7 or web-based protocol as the standard to be used. To overcome the problems imposed by the existing HIS parts, the SIGIC Board decided that the HIS strategic plan has to be defined to fit the mission statement. All the relevant stakeholders must be involved. Therefore a stakeholder-oriented approach was preferred to cope with the complexity of the problem. Considering the Regional Health Authorities (that could speak in the name of the hospitals) objectives, three task forces teams were defined to address those objectives: Clinical decision-making information system; Management information system; and Networking and Data warehouse. To manage each of these groups was defined a co-ordinator from the SIGIC team. Each workgroup defined the policies within their area of responsibility, prioritised projects and allocated budgets. To address the strategic planning, that would support the HIS, the Winter at al. (2001) methodology was adapted, comprising "the health unit strategic goals assessment", "the identification of the current state of the HIS" and "an analysis on how far the current information system fits the goals". The methodology for a strategic HIS plan encompasses the following five steps:

a.   Strategic goals of SIGIC (MS, 2005);
b.   Description of the hospitals surgery-related IS current state;
c.   Analysis and assessment of the current state of the HIS (MS, 2005);

d. Description of the planned state of the SIGLIC (MS, 2005);

e. Roadmap definition: Path from the current to the planned state: This plan assigned resources and concrete deadlines (although flexible) for partial results, as well as assigning priorities to individual tasks and the dependencies between tasks. Representatives of the different stakeholders were involved in the definition of the future state process.

5.2 System selection and implementation leadership strategy

The IS integration is usually a very difficult task due to the complexity and the number of different systems involved. An integration process can be technically accomplished through two different ways by means of a direct link or by means of message exchange (Lenz & Kuhn, 2002). Since the HIS is composed by many different suppliers, following a "best-of-breed" approach, it was advisable to opt for the second one. An additional assumption was defined: the message exchange system will have to be web-based. The freedom to exchange some of the applications in the near future was among the criteria considered. A good communication infrastructure is essential so that it ensures in all cases messages to be correctly delivered to the addressees in the proper sequence and that standard message protocols are used: the solution proposed implied the utilisation of Virtual Private Network within the Ministry of Health private network.

There are several advantages in adopting a phased implementation strategy (Spil et al., 1999). Moreover phasing the implementation would allow for a better financial resources management, as time delay would diminish considerably the financial risk. Phasing is also the best way to address learning, because one can learn with early projects and adopt new measures in the following ones thus augmenting the probability of fitting with the users' requirements and therefore diminishing the risk of failure. The development of subsystems or changes in existing systems was carefully planned within a finite period of time but allowing some flexibility due to financial restrictions. Decisions on budget and personnel allocations must be made, and priorities in relation to other, competing projects must be set. One must also understand the introduction of IS imposes changes on an organisation process. SIGIC program implies that surgeons (anaesthetists, nurses and other technicians) will work after the normal daily schedule. This additional work will be like another service provided by the hospital. The volume of activity of SIGIC in a hospital can be paramount, eventually creating the need to hire, or reallocate, a manager just focusing on SIGIC activities.

Organisations usually follow several stages in their growth toward a situation in which information systems are fully integrated. Nolan (1979) growth model was used to address maturity of hospital IS understanding. Galliers & Sutherland (1991) observed that most organisations overtake maturity stages one by one, and that the transformation into the formalisation and maturity stages especially requires explicit leadership by managers. At most hospitals, the next Nolan stage implied the rethinking and redesign of the whole organisational structure that support SIGIC.

5.3 The process of selection of a HIS solution

The selection process was developed through a set of test prototypes to reduce both risks and the strategic gap. To support the selection decision-making process an operational methodology was used. Like SMARTER (Graeber, 2001) or the TRIDENT (Tavares, 1984) both allow for a balanced approach. In the TRIDENT Methodology the problem is addressed with a five-phase process balanced by three parameters (quality, cost and implementation time):

Phase 1 – Needs Assessment and Planning;
Phase 2 – Gathering Information;
Phase 3 – Vendor Demonstrations;
Phase 4 – Negotiation;
Phase 5 – Pilot Projects implementation.

The process analysis considered the technology supplier's that responded to the call. One pilot projects was selected to be implemented in Alentejo and Algarve region.

When defining a HIS, one must also consider its time evolution. Whatever the Information System considered it will need, sooner or later, an up-grade or maintenance. Recent trends enhance the importance of processes, workflow management and web-based applications as best practice (Lenz & Kuhn, 2002). With these conditions satisfied, the hospitals in the pilot test could then proceed towards the HIS. The initial analysis and diagnosis of the IS concluded that: a) The hospitals' IS are very complex system, with several different sub-systems and different actors; b) Most application were not linked and coherently integrated together. There were in fact only few point-to-point connections between applications from the same supplier; c) Enormous difficulty accessing timely precise information; d) Some problems regarding specific applications due to lack of knowledge and a troubled dependency from technology suppliers; e) Difficulties in correctly training the healthcare professionals. Theses conclusions and department objectives were considered at a workshop that defined the roadmap.

The idea is to give to surgeons an information system that allows them to make decisions and therefore adds value. So he/she can become somewhat positively dependent on the use of the system. With valid data the mangers might gain as far as possible a clear perspective over the surgeon's behaviour as he/she writes orders to allocate resources. This sort of resources-use control is desirable as it allows a highly autonomous group of professionals to allocate resources according to a specific best practice available with the system. Although one must recognise that this is a dramatic change in the relationship between managers and health professionals that need proper leadership. The option for the "integrator" had in mind the efficiency and clinical gains in the communications between applications, i.e. the benefits for patient service itself. The future implementation of an electronic patient record system also needs the support of the integrator, in order to combine all the data that is needed to sustain the increasing demand for quality, alert and clinical knowledge systems and, if possible, clinical decision-support systems. It is usually unsuccessful to implement a electronic clinical system without guarantying integration beforehand.

The methodology followed a Roadmap framework, which allowed associating both SIGIC and hospitals' HIS strategy. The added value to SIGIC is clearly shown by the appropriated budget allocation for the investment needed to build the information system that will help healthcare professionals to serve the patients better. There was also a clear advantage in parallel process development because each task force could either develop them individually without depending on the others or address difficulties independently. The roadmap had the objective of mapping the short-medium term strategy into actions (Kuperman, 2000). It was also given special attention to the users and to the decision making processes by the setting up of a workshop, which was based on the definition of management indicators that would cope with the SIGIC strategy.

6. Improving the access to surgery with SIGLIC information system

SIGLIC is the information system defined to support real time exchange of information of all the SIGIC decision-making processes. The knowledge is integrated with a unified and coherent set of information. This information is based on the data model required to perform the management of waiting list for surgery. By integrating the production processes, while generating cost and value, it will culminate in the perception of the gains in health and the value perceived by the patient.

The Information model includes the following items: information on patients and events to allow "Process management", "clinical information" for "Disease Management" and "financial data" to allow the "Contract management" between the health units, from which data is gathered to improve access management (quality treatment, i.e. gains in health, and value perceived for the patient). The information should be recorded by hospitals (with the responsibility for the information contents) in accordance with a set of standards and then integrated into the central database of SIGIC. It was also clearly defined who would produce and sign the information, the minimal data set (standardized information), and all the information to be recorded is to be included in the workflow.

The quality of the integrated information from the hospitals is guaranteed by a set of tools that validate its consistency, and rejects non-compliant data. The information is recorded in hospitals throughout the process of managing the patient on WLS and integrated daily in the central database (Figure 3).

SIGLIC - Process of acquiring the information

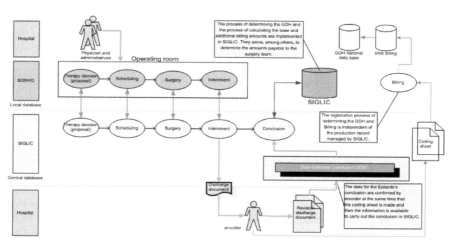

The information is recorded in hospitals throughout the process of managing the patient on WLS and integrated daily in the central database.

Fig. 3. Flow of information between hospitals and the central database.

The information exchanges between hospitals and central database are executed (two-way) daily. They must be subject to central data sync with the hospitals and to a reporting system for errors that identifies gaps in the transaction. Thus the central IS does not create parallel processes but generates an integrated knowledge of hospital activity with only 24 hours of delay. In SIGIC, all the information campaigns, the training sessions for professionals and the provision of quality information are key measures to promote the participation of all stakeholders in this process of improvement.

7. Results: Improving the access to surgery from 2000 to 2010

7.1 The SIGIC evolution

The SIGIC system was defined in 2003 and started operating in June the first 2004 as a pilot project in the region of Algarve and Alentejo. The regions that followed were Lisbon, the Tagus Valley and North on the first of June 2005. The last region to join was Centre on first October 2005.The Centre region's entrance in the SIGIC system (with SIGLIC) was somewhat delayed because of technical integration problems on a set of hospitals information systems whose software versions were not compatible with the SIGIC (Palmeira, 2010). In 2007, three years after being on service, the number of patients waiting for a surgery was of 234.463 (TDC, 2007). Comparing this number with the first semester of 2009 (169.461 (and from 175.761 in December 2008), an additional reduction in the number of patients waiting for surgery was obtained. The median of waiting time (TE) at the WLS was 3,4 months in June 2009 (a reduction from 3,7 months in December 08), in spite of the increase in number of patients entering the WLS (+7,1%), first semester of 2008.

The Accounting Tribunal report criticizes SIGIC for not showing management indicators regarding productivity and the hospital units capacity, which would enable a higher management efficiency regarding surgery production and the number of surgeries produced per specialty (TDC, 2007). Recently, the program e-SIGIC was developed. This innovation enables each patient to Access to the WLS and check about His/her position in the list, and therefore knowing the waiting time for surgery. This Web-based program started to operate on December 2009, which allowed for the improvement of communication with patients and easing their access to relevant information using internet.

7.2 Evolution of the performance indicators on WLS

The SIGIC program results are very positive (Figure 4, 5, 6 and 7) and show clearly the importance of developing an information systems that allows improved resources allocation. Figure 4. shows the number of people in waiting list for surgery has decreased 33.7%, which is an evidence that the system is actually working. The impact could also be translated in reduction time: the waiting time for surgery decreased from 8.6 to 3.4 months, meaning a 60.5% reduction simply being allowed through better system organization and management (Figure 5.). At the same time, this improvement has allowed an increase on patient's entrance (meaning an improvement in accessibility to surgery) from 426,949 to 560,695 episodes (+31.3%) (Figure 6.). This was possible because of an increase on scheduled surgery from 345,321 to 475,293 episodes (+37.6%) has been provided (Figure 7.). Another significant impact has been on hospital transfer (a usual bureaucratic process) which has increased from 3,003 to 38,976 episodes (+1200%). This last result shows the real impact of an integrated IS over bureaucracy. Should be noted, that some of the decrease in number of

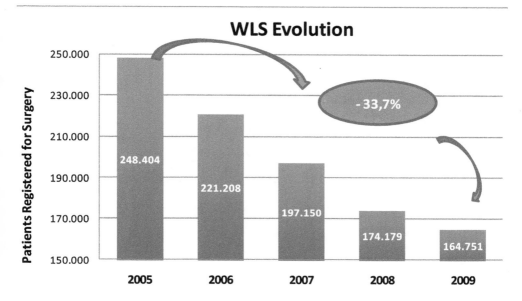

Fig. 4. Waiting list for surgery time evolution.

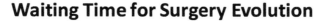

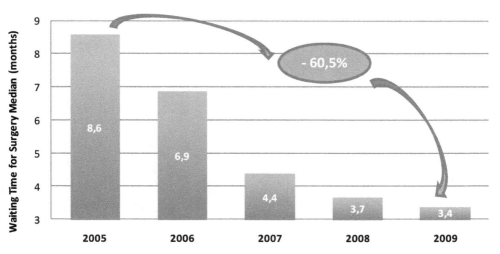

Fig. 5. Waiting time to surgery reduction.

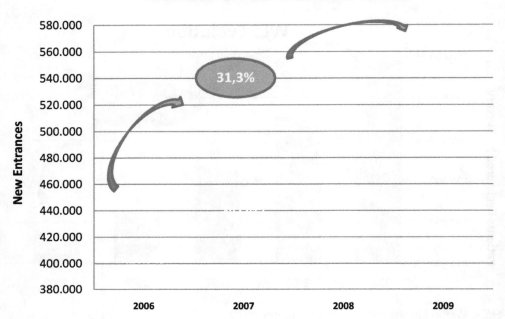

Fig. 6. The evolution of new patient entrances to the waiting surgery list.

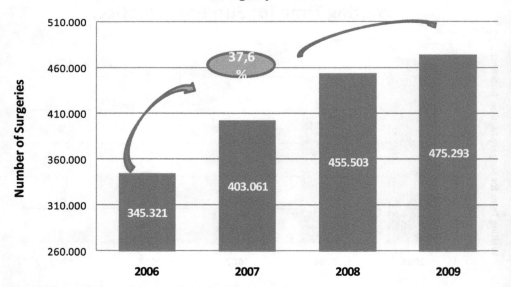

Fig. 7. The evolution of the number of surgeries performed.

patients waiting was due to systematic purge to the list, identifying those already operated, already deceased, enrolled in more than one list, no longer indicated for surgery or non traceable. This effect was felt mostly during the early years and does not overpower the system´s actual measured increase in efficiency.

8. Debate: The positives and the negatives

From the case presented one should conclude that SIGLIC, the IS that supports SIGIC, has been essential to ensure the delivery of benefits to the patient and healthcare providers in improving the access to surgery. The results are quite impressive, deriving from a professional application of IS design and implementation principles that allowed the overcoming of communication barriers and the lack of operating rooms management practices.

The SIGLIC system enabled the SIGIC program to cover the whole country and furthermore, allowed many hospitals to increase the participation of surgeons and a more efficient usage of operating rooms. This is only part of a wider effort to implement a comprehensive strategy to consistently allow information collection and sharing within Portuguese healthcare sector to improve resources' usage management. Future work would include both the analysis of the use of the IS itself and of the actual health gains provided with the surgeries.

From Siciliani & Hurst (2004) we know that, on the supply side, evidence suggests that both capacity and financial incentives towards productivity can play an important role (as SIGIC can also prove). And on the demand side, the SIGIC also induced the raising of clinical thresholds with significant reduction of waiting times but with an increment in the tension between clinicians and policy makers.

9. Conclusion

This chapter describes the design and first results of the use of an information system (SIGLIC) supporting the integrated management program (SIGA) to improve the access to surgery in Portugal. SIGIC, the Ministry of Health's agency responsible for access to surgery management, started re-thinking the system in 2005 by re-defining key processes and workflows.

Although the focus was on improving the access equality, the Portuguese Accounting Tribunal has released recently (second semester 2009) that, according to its criteria, these equity principles were not met, once there are still patients referred to the private and social sectors, which are not part of the WSL and do not hold the same warranties and rights (TOC, 2009).

The designed information system SIGLIC integrates all hospitals with surgery with every other hospital, where it picks data to allow the search for optimal solutions for each patient. In the context of SIGIC (Waiting List for Surgery's Integrated Management System) "access" means to assure the treatment by services in terms of quality, standards, equity, process and transparency.

SIGIC's goals are to reduce waiting time for surgery, to apply identical standards to all patients, to benefit from good use of resources and, to create a national structure of homogeneous information based in a system of data collection. The methodology followed was to: a) "survey of information systems and technology in Demand/Supply/Resources"; b) "institutionalization and monitoring of procedural standards for management of the Waiting List for Surgery (WLS)", c) provide "evaluation by results" and, d) "Correction of deviations to the standard". To fulfill SIGIC's objectives a management model (SIGA) and SIGLIC were created as to support it. By now 57 public hospitals and 96 private clinics and hospitals (with convention in SIGIC) have joined the SIGIC network.

The Information model includes the following items: information on patients and events to allow "Process management", "clinical information" for "Disease Management" and "financial data" to allow management between the health units, from which data is gathered, to improve access management. The information is recorded by hospitals in accordance with a set of standards and integrated into the central database of SIGIC.

The quality of integrated information from the hospitals is guaranteed by a set of tools to validate its consistency, rejecting non-compliant data. The information is recorded in hospitals throughout the process of managing the patients on WLS and integrated daily in the central database. The results since 2005 show the importance of an integrated information system to overcome the bureaucracy: There was a 36% improvement in number of scheduled surgical episodes and 60% reduction in days on waiting time.

At the present moment SIGIC has almost all its core and support applications. If all these applications were working properly they would be guarantying the efficiency of the Hospital's productive process further.

Future research includes understanding regional differences and benchmark better practices in prioritizing and managing the WLS. Regarding the SIGLIC, there is still space for improvements: the development of alert systems and of mechanisms to enhance the participation of the patients in the process.

10. Acknowledgment

We would like to thanks to Dr. Pedro Gomes (M.D.), the Director of SIGIC program of the Ministry of Health for fruitful discussion and valuable information; and to Dr. Carla Nunes (M.D.), orthopedic surgeon, for helpful advices and discussion.

11. References

Banta, D. & Wija, O. (2000) Introduction: Health Technology Assessment and the European Union. *International Journal of Technology Assessment in Health Care* 16(2): 299-302.
Carr, T., Teucher, U., Mann, J. & Casson, A.G. (2009) Waiting for surgery from the patient perspective. Psychology Research and Behavior Management 2: 107-119.
Cromwell DA, Griffiths DA, Kreis IA (2002) Surgery dot.com: the quality of information disseminated by Web-based waiting time information services. *Med J Aust.* 177(5): 253-5.
Dexter, F., Macario, A. & Traub, R.D. (2000) Enterprise-wide patient scheduling information systems to coordinate surgical clinic and operating room scheduling can impair operating room efficiency. *Anesth Analg* 91: 617-26.

EOHSP (2009) European Observatory on Health Systems and Policies: http://www.euro.who.int/observatory (assessed on the 14th of November 2009).

Glaser, J. P. & Salzberg, C. (2011) *The Strategic Application of IT in the Healthcare Organizations*, Jossey Bass (third edition).

Galliers, R. D., & Sutherland A. R. (1991) Information systems management and strategy formulation: the 'stages of growth' model revisited. *Journal of Information Systems*, 1:2.

Gauld, R. & Derrett, S. (2000) Solving the surgical waiting list problems? New Zealand's "booking system" *Int J Health Plann Mgmt* 15:259-72.

GoSA (2006) *Policy Framework and Associated Procedural Guidelines for Elective Surgery Services*. Department of Health. Government of South Australia.

GoSA (2003) *Policy for the Management of Elective Surgical Admissions in Metropolitan Public Hospitals*. Department of Health. Government of South Australia.

Graeber, S. (2001) How to Select a Clinical Information System, *AMIA*.

Grilo A, Lapão LV, Gonçalves RJ, Cruz-Machado V. (2009) "The Development of Interoperability Strategies in Health Organizations", chapter accept to be included in the forthcoming book: *Handbook of Business Information Systems*, World Scientific Publishing.

Hasselbring, W., Peterson, R., Smits, M., Spanjers, M. & Strate R. (2000) Strategic Information Management for a Dutch University Hospital. *Stud Health Technol Inform*. 77:885-9.

Haugen, H. & Woodside, J.R. (2010) *Beyond Implementation: Prescribing for lasting EMR adoption*. Magnusson Skor.

Kim, S.C. & Horowitz, I. (2002) Scheduling hospital services: the efficacy of elective-surgery quotas. Omega 30(5): 335-346.

Kuhn, K. A. Giuse, D.A., Lapão, L.V., & Wurst, S.H.R. (2007) Expanding the Scope of Health Information Systems: From Hospitals to Regional Networks, to National Infrastructures, and Beyond. *Methods of Information in Medicine* 46(4): 500-2.

Iversen, T. (1993) A theory of hospital waiting lists. *Journal of Health Economics* 12(1): 55-71

Jeston, J. & Nelis, J. (2006) *Business Process Management. Practical Guidelines to Successful Implementations*. Butterworth-Heinemann, Elsevier.

Kuperman GJ, Spurr C, Flamnimini S, Bates D, Glaser J (2000) A Clinical Information Systems Strategy for a Large Integrated Delivery Network. *AMIA 2000 Conference Proceedings*, 1067:438-442.

Lapão, LV. (2007) Survey on the Status of the Hospital Information Systems in Portugal, *Methods of Information in Medicine*, 46 4: 493-499.

Lapão LV, Rebuge A, Mira-da-Silva M, Gomes R (2009). ITIL Assessment in a Healthcare Environment: The Role of IT Governance at Hospital S. Sebastião. Studies in Health Technology and Informatics Vol. 150

Lapão LV & Dussault G (2011). "PACES: a National leadership program in support of Primary-Care Reform in Portugal". Leadership in Health Services. 24: 295 – 307.

Lenz R and Kuhn KA. (2002) Integration of Heterogeneous and Autonomous Systems in Hospitals. *Business Briefing*: Data Management & Storage Technology.

McKee, M & Healy, J (2002) *Hospitals in a Changing Europe*. Open University Press.

MS (1999) Healthcare in Portugal: A Strategy for a new Century 1998-2002. Ministry of Health (in Portuguese).

MS (2004) Presidência do Conselho de Ministros, *Resolução do Conselho de Ministros n°79/2004*, Lisboa: Diário da Républica N°147, I Série-B (published on the 24th June).

MS (2005) *Manual de Gestão de Inscritos para Cirurgia*. Processo de Gestão do Utente (Manual SIGIC), Unidade Central de Gestão de Inscritos para Cirurgia, Ministério da Saúde.

MS (2011) *Dados do Serviço Nacional de Saúde*. Ministério da Saúde.

Nolan, R. (1979) The Crisis in Data Processing. *Havard Business Revie* Mar-Apr, 115.

Palmeira, C. (2010) A Equidade no Acesso à Saúde: A problemática do sistema integrado de gestão de inscritos para cirurgia. *Tese de mestrado integrado em Medicina*. FMUP.

Porter, M.E. & Teisberg E.O. (2006) *Redefining Health Care: Creating Value-Based Competition on Results*, Harvard Business School Press: Boston.

PRLD (2007) SIGIC Law. Law 41/2007 of 24th of August, article 3rd . *Portuguese Republic Law Diary* (In Portuguese).

TDC (2007) *Relatório n° 25/07 -2ª.S, Processo n° 50/05*. AUDIT. Tribunal de Contas de Portugal.

TDC (2009) *Relatório sobre SIGIC*. (30th July 2009). Tribunal de Contas de Portugal.

Sibbald, S. L., Singer P. A., Upshur, R. & Martin, D.K. Priority setting: what constitutes success? A conceptual framework for successful priority setting. *BMC Health Services Research* 9(43): 1-12.

Siciliani, L. & Hurst, J. (2005) Tackling excessive waiting times for elective surgery: a comparative analysis of policies in 12 OECD countries. *Health Policy* 72 (2005): 201-215.

Smaltz, D.H., Glaser J.P, Skinner, R.I. and Cunningham T.T. (2005) The CEO-CIO Partnership: Harnessing the value of information technology in Healthcare. *Healthcare Information Manangement Systems Society*.

Spil, T., Meeberg, H. & Sikkel K. (1999) The definition, selection and the implementation of a new hospital information system to prepare the hospital for the electronic future: an example of a project based education. *Proceedings of the 32nd Hawaii International Conference on System Sciences*.

Tavares, L.V. (1984) "The TRIDENT approach to rank alternative tenders for large engineering projects", Foundations of Control Engineering.

Valente, R., Testi, A., Tanfani, E., Fato, M., Porro, I., Santo, M., Santori, G., Torre, G. & Ansaldo, G. (2009) A model to prioritize access to elective surgery on the basis of clinical urgency and waiting time. *BMC Health Services Research* 9(1)

van Ackere, A. & Smith, P. C. (1999) Towards a macro model of National Health Service waiting lists. System Dynamics Review, *Special Issue: Health and Health Care Dynamics*. 15 (3): 225-252.

VanBerkel, P.T. & Blake, J.T. (2007) A comprehensive simulation for wait time reduction and capacity planning applied in general surgery. *Health Care Management Science* 10 (4): 373-385

Winter, A.F. et al; Strategic Information Management Plans: the basis for systematic information management in hospitals, *International Journal of Medical Informatics* 64 (2001) 99-109.

Winter, A.P. et al; Purpose and Structure of Strategic Plans for Information Management in Hospitals. *Medical Infobahn for Europe*. Amsterdam: IOS Press. S. 880-884.

Part 2

Bioinformatics Methods

3

A Comprehensive Analysis of MALDI-TOF Spectrometry Data

Malgorzata Plechawska-Wojcik
Lublin University of Technology,
Poland

1. Introduction

Today, biology and medicine need developed technologies and bioinformatics methods. Effective methods of analysis combine different technologies and can operate on many levels. Multi-step analysis needs to be performed to get information helpful in diagnosis or medical treatment tasks. All those processing needs the informatics approach to bioinformatics, proteomics and knowledge discovery methods.

Scientists find proteomic data difficult to analyse. On the other hand, the proteomic analysis of tissues like blood, plasma and urine might have an invaluable contribution to biological and medical research. They seem to be an alternative way of searching for new diagnostic methods, medical treatment and drug development. For example, typical analytical methods have problems with dealing with cancer diseases. Proteomics is a promising approach to those issues.

Proteomic signals carry an enormous amount of data. They reflect whole sequences of proteins responsible for various life processes of the organism. This diversity of data makes it hard to find specific information about, for example, the severity of the cancer. To discover interesting knowledge researchers need to combine a variety of techniques. One of the basic methods of tissue analysis is mass spectrometry. This technique measures the mass-to-charge ratio of charged particles.

There are various types of mass spectrometry techniques. They differ in the types of ion source and mass analysers. The MALDI-TOF (Coombes et al., 2007) is a technique widely applicable in proteomic research. The MALDI (Matrix - Assisted Laser Desorption / Ionisation) is a soft ionisation technique and the TOF (time of flight) is a detector determining the mass of ions. Samples are mixed with a highly absorbent matrix and bombarded with a laser. The matrix stimulates the process of transforming laser energy into excitation energy (Morris et al., 2005). After this process analyte molecules are sputtered and spared. The mass of ions is determined on the basis of time particular ions take to drift through the spectrometer. Velocities and intensities of ions obtained in such a way (Morris et. al., 2005) are proportional to the mass-to-charge (m/z) ratio.

The analysis of mass spectrometry data is a complex task (Plechawska 2008a; Plechawska 2008b). The process of gaining biological information and knowledge from raw data is composed of several steps. A proper mass spectrometry data analysis requires creating and solving a model and estimating its parameters (Plechawska 2008a). There are many types of models and methods which might be used. All of them, however, include mass spectrum preprocessing, which need to to be done before the general analysis. Preprocessing methods need be adjusted to data. Spectra have some noise levels which need to be removed. Denoising and baseline corrections are done to get rid of the noise which might be caused by spectrometer inaccuracy or by sample contamination. Also, normalisation should be performed. After these steps, peak detection and quantification can be done. Successful preprocessing is a condition of reliable mass spectrometry data analysis (Coombes et. al., 2007). All elements of the mass spectral analysis are closely related. Any performed operation has an influence on the further quality of results. Not only the set of methods and parameters is important. The proper order of methods also matters.

There is an extensive literature on mass spectrum analysis problems (Plechawska et al., 2011). One can find several techniques of peak detection and identification. A very popular approach is to use local maxima and minima. Such methods (Morris et. al., 2005; Yasui et. al., 2003; Tibshirani et. al., 2004) usually compare local maxima with noise level. There are also methods (Zhang et al., 2007) considering the signal to noise ratio. This ratio needs to be high enough to identify a true peak with a local maximum. Such methods choose peaks with the highest intensities. Similar ideas (Mantini et al., 2007; Mantini et al., 2008) consider using predefined thresholds depending on the noise level. Peak detection is usually done on denoised spectra. Moreover, intervals based on local maxima and minima are calculated. Constituent intervals have differences between the height of the maxima and minima found. In addition, using the mean spectrum was proposed (Coombes et. al., 2007). Other methods (Fung & Enderwick, 2002) use regions which are determined to enable easier peak detection based on the signal to noise ratio. Peaks need to have an large enough area and appropriate width, which depends on starting and ending points of peaks and valleys on both sides of the apex. Peaks may be also considered a continuous range of points where intensities are high enough (Eidhammer et al., 2007). Another approach is using peak clusters to find peaks of the highest intensities (Zhang et al., 2007). There are also methods which try to distinguish true peaks from noise and contaminants. Du et al. (Du et al., 2006) for example use the shape of peaks. Some methods consider the mass spectrometer resolution. There are also methods turning spectrum decomposition into the sum of their constituent functions (Randolph et al., 2005) or the sum of the Levy processes (Zhang et al., 2007).

2. Mass spectrum modelling

Before the main decomposition, preprocessing needs to be performed. In our analysis we apply the following methods:

- Trimming is the cutting of the lower and/or upper parts of spectra according to specified boundaries designated by the type of analysis.
- Binning with a defined mask is a technique reducing the number of data points in a single spectrum. The researcher has to keep in mind that this process additionally gives noise reduction. This is optional method. It should be used if the number of the spectrum data points is too large to perform efficient calculations.
- Interpolation is a process which may be defined as the unification of measurements points along the m/z axes. It is needed in the case of dealing with a data set of spectra. Unification is obligatory if all spectra are to be analysed simultaneously.

- Baseline correction is an essential part of preprocessing. Baseline is a special type of noise which needs to be removed. It represents a systematic artifact formed by a cloud of matrix molecules hitting the detector (Morris et al., 2005). This noise is seen in the early part of the spectrum. Among typical methods of baseline correction one can find a simple frame with fixed sizes and quantilles. Our experience shows that a simple frame with the appropriate size is good enough.
- Smoothing and noise reduction might be performed in several ways. One can use wavelet transformation (for example the widely-used undecimated discrete-wavelet transformation, UDWT), the least-squares digital polynomial filter (Savitzky and Golay filters) or nonparametric smoothing (locally-weighted linear regression with specified window size and type of kernel). In our analysis we usually make use of a polynomial filter. However it is also possible to skip noise reduction due to the specificity of the decomposition method.
- Normalisation is an important preprocessing method consisting in minimising differences between spectra and thier peak intensities. The most popular methods are scaling all spectra to total ion current (TIC) value or to constant noise. We found the TIC value appropriate for our analysis. It is calculated as the area under the curve, usually using the trapezoidal method.
- The mean spectrum calculation is useful in analysing data sets containing many mass spectra of the same type. The mean spectrum facilitating the simultaneous analysis of all spectra. Even small peaks are usually detected during mean spectrum analysis. Finding peaks in the mean spectrum are regarded as even more sensitive (Morris et al., 2005).

Most preprocessing steps need to be conducted under the supervision of the user. The parameters of the baseline correction especially need to be adjusted to the data. The order of operations is fixed. Many research studies were conducted in this area and this order has become a standard over the past few years. Some of operations might be skipped - but it should be depended on the data.

2.1 Gaussian mixture model decomposition

Our method of spectrum analysis is based on Gaussian Mixture decomposition. The Gaussian Mixture Model (GMM) (Everitt & Hand, 1981) with the appropriate number of components is suitable for spectrum modelling because they also might be used for noise modelling and determining. The idea of using GMM is that one peak is represented by a single distribution (Plechawska-Wojcik, 2011a). All peaks and the noise are represented by the mixture model. A mixture model is a combination of a finite number of distributions. The number of components might be estimated by the Bayesian Information Criterion (BIC).

The fitting is done with the Expectation-Maximisation algorithm (EM) performing maximising the likelihood function. A typical mixture model is a combination of a finite number of probability distributions (eq. 1).

$$f^{mix}(x, \alpha_1, ..., \alpha_K, p_1, ..., p_K) = \sum_{k=1}^{K} \alpha_k f_k(x, p_k) \qquad (1)$$

where K is the number of components in the mixture and $\alpha_k, k = 1, 2, ... K$ are weights of the

particular component, $\sum_{k=1}^{K} \alpha_k = 1$. The Gaussian distribution is given with two parameters:

mean μ_k and standard deviation σ_k.

The Expectation-Maximisation (EM) algorithm (Dempster et al., 1977) is a nonlinear method and is composed of two main steps performed in a loop. The expectation step (E) consists of the calculation of the distribution of hidden variables (eq. 2).

$$p(k \mid x_n, p^{old}) = \frac{\alpha_k^{old} f_k(x_n, p^{old})}{\sum_{\kappa=1}^{K} \alpha_k^{old} f_k(x_n, p^{old})} \qquad (2)$$

The maximisation step (M) calculates new mixture parameter values. Formulas adjusted to mass spectrometry data are given by (eq. 3).

$$\mu_k^{new} = \frac{\sum_{n=1}^{N} x_n y_n p(k \mid x_n, p_{old})}{\sum_{n=1}^{N} p(k \mid x_n, p_{old}) y_n}, k = 1, 2, ..., K$$

$$(\sigma_k^{new})^2 = \frac{\sum_{n=1}^{N} (x_n - \mu_k^{new})^2 p(k \mid x_n, p_{old})}{\sum_{n=1}^{N} p(k \mid x_n, p_{old}) y_n}, k = 1, 2, ..., K \qquad (3)$$

$$\alpha_k^{new} = \frac{\sum_{n=1}^{N} p(k \mid x_n, p^{old}) y_n}{N}$$

The calculated means represent the M/Z values of peaks, whereas standard deviations indicate the widths of peaks. Weights determine the shares of particular peaks in the spectrum. This method may be applied to individual spectra or to the mean spectrum calculated from the data set. In the case of the mean spectrum, the obtained means and standard deviations are treated as, respectively, M/Z values and widths of peaks in every single spectrum of the data set. The weights are calculated separately for each spectrum. The simple least-squares method might be used to obtain those weights.

Examples of a mass spectra collection analysis are presented in Fig.1. Fig.1a,c present the results of our calculations for single spectra with 40 components and Fig.1b,d presents the results with the use of the mean spectrum. The mean spectrum is presented in Fig.2.

2.2 Parameters of the decomposition process

There are several aspects which need to be considered before the decomposition. The first is the number of components which needs to be known before carrying out the analysis. The best solution is to use one of the available criteria. These are BIC (the Bayesian Information Criterion), AIC (the Akaike Information Criterion), ICOMP (the Information Complexity Criterion), AWE (the Approximate Weight of Evidence), MIR (the Minimum Information Ratio) and NEC (the Normalised Entropy Criterion). The proper number of components should minimise (or for some criteria maximise) the value of the chosen criterion. Most of

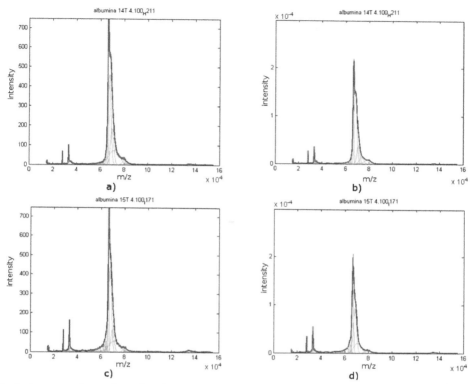

Fig. 1. A comparison of results obtained with and without the mean spectrum.

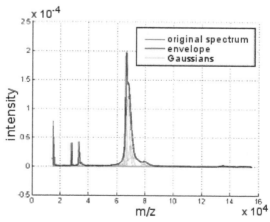

Fig. 2. The mean spectrum.

the mentioned criteria are based on the likelihood function. We chose the BIC criterion because it is easy to calculate and it considers such parameters as the size of the sample and the value of the likelihood function. Formulas defining the mentioned criteria are presented in Tab1. In the presented formulas models the parameters are marked as ψ .

The main disadvantage of using criteria to estimate the number of components is the fact that it is a time-consuming method. A single use of each criterion gives a result for the single number of components. To obtain reliable results the calculations need to be repeated many times for each single number of components. The example of using the BIC criterion for data presented in Fig.1 and Fig.2 is shown in Fig.3. According to Fig.3, the BIC criterion needs to be maximised. Results stabilise for 40 components, so this number was considered to be appropriate for the further analysis.

There are also different ways of dealing with the unknown number of the components problem. It is possible to use different, simple method of peak detection. Such methods work fast, because they are based on local maxima and minima. However, it is a reliable method only in the case of spectra which do not have many overlapped peaks.

Criterions	Formulas
BIC (the Bayesian Information Criterion) (Schwarz, 1978)	$BIC(g) = 2\log L(\hat{\psi}) - d\log n$
AIC (the Akaike Information Criterion) (Akaike, 1974)	$AIC(g) = -2\log L(\hat{\psi}) + 2d$
ICOMP (the Information Complexity Criterion) (Bozdogan, 1993; Bozdogan, 1990)	$ICOMP(g) = -2\log L(\hat{\psi}) + C_1 - C_2$ $C_1 = d\log[d^{-1} \sum\limits_{i=1}^{g} \{\pi_i^{-1} tr\hat{\Sigma}_i + \frac{1}{2}tr(\hat{\Sigma}_i\hat{\Sigma}) + \frac{1}{2}tr(\hat{\Sigma}_i)^2 + \sum\limits_{v=1}^{P} (\hat{\Sigma}_i)^2_{vv}\}]$ $C_2 = (p+2)\sum\limits_{i=1}^{g} \log(|\hat{\Sigma}_i|) - p\sum\limits_{v=1}^{P} \log(n\hat{\pi}_i) + gp\log(2n)$ $d = gp + \frac{1}{2}gp(p+1)$
AWE (the Approximate Weight of Evidence) (Banfield & Raftery, 1993)	$AWE(g) = -2\log L_C + 2d(3/2 + \log n)$
MIR (the Minimum Information Ratio) (Windham & Cutler, 1993)	$MIR(g) = 1 - \left\| \psi^{m+1} - \psi^m \right\| / \left\| \psi^m - \psi^{m-1} \right\|$
NEC (the Normalized Entropy Criterion) (Celeux & Soromenho, 1996)	$NEC(g) = \dfrac{EN(\hat{r})}{\log L(\hat{\psi}) - \log L(\hat{\psi}*)}$

Table 1. Criteria used to estimate the number of components.

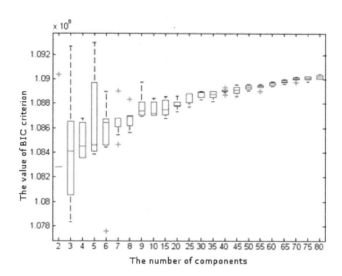

Fig. 3. The estimation of the number of components using BIC criterion.

It is also possible to reduce the number of components during calculations. This correction is based on the values of probabilities calculated during the M step of the EM procedure. If they are too small (very close to 0) it usually means that the number of components is overstated. Essential support is also given by the model testing procedure. EM calculations might be suspended after a few iterations. The researcher can check the so-far obtained weights and means indicating the peak localisations. If he/she finds many very small weights, or means are found to be located very close to each other, it usually means that the number of specified components is too large. Suspending the EM procedure makes sense because of the characteristic of the algorithm. It converges very fast at the beginning and after that it slows down. That is why the checking of the results after 10-20 calculations fairy well illustrates the quality of the modelling.

The other aspect which needs to be considered is the generation of initial parameters values. The EM algorithm is sensitive to the initial values. If they are poorly chosen, the quality of calculations might not be reliable. One option is to randomise them from the appropriate distribution. The better one, however, is to use the simple method of peak detection. This method gives less biased, more reliable results. The important thing is to add small Gaussian arousals to the results obtained from the peak-detection method.

The next decomposition aspect to be mentioned is the stop criterion. According our simulations one good idea is to use a stop criterion based on the likelihood value (eq. 4) and the maximum likelihood rule (eq. 5). The maximum likelihood rule states that the higher value of the likelihood function, the better the parameters estimation can be gained. Using the maximum likelihood rule gives the certainty of stability because of monotonicity of the likelihood function (Fig. 4).

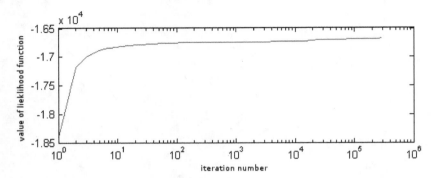

Fig. 4. The monotinicity of the likelihood rule.

$$L(p,x) = L(p) = f(x_1, x_2, ..., x_N, p) = \prod_{n=1}^{N} f(x_n, p) \qquad (4)$$

$$\hat{p} = \arg\max \prod_{n=1}^{N} f(x_n, p) \qquad (5)$$

Maximum likelihood itself is an efficient method of parameters estimation. However, it cannot be used in the problem of spectral decomposition. The problem consists in the fact that we do not know the assignment of the Gaussians to the respective peaks. The EM algorithm deals with it using hidden variables. The probabilities of assignment are calculated in each iteration and finally the right assignment is found.

The decomposition with the EM algorithm is slower than using simple methods based on local minima and maxima. However, it copes better with spectra containing overlapped peaks. There are many examples of spectra which cannot be solved by such typical methods. Examples of decomposed spectra obtained from different methods are presented in Fig. 5.

The next argument for Gaussian decomposition is that using an EM algorithm and a mean spectrum eliminates the necessity for alignment procedure processing. This operation is done to align detected peaks among all spectra in the dataset. Those mismatches are due to measurement errors. The alignment procedure needs to be performed on most of peak processing procedures. It is a hard and difficult process. EM decomposition is based on the assumption that peaks are covered with Gaussians defined by means and standard deviations. That is why the m/z values do not need to match exactly to Gaussians means – we accept slight differences between peaks among different spectra in the dataset.

The method discussed in this chapter is based on Gaussian distributions. However, it is also possible to use different distributions, like Poisson, log-normal or beta. High-resolution spectra contain asymmetric peaks with the right skewedness. In such cases it is a good idea to use log-normal or beta distributions (Guindani et al., 2006). MALDI-ToF spectra are low-resolution and there is no skewedness seen. That is why Gaussian distributions are more appropriate to use. The second reason we use Gaussian distributions is connected with the error of the spectrometer measurement. This noise can be modelled in a natural way with Gaussians.

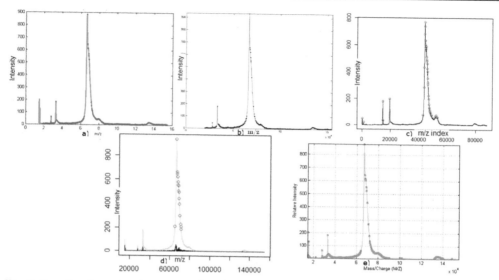

Fig. 5. Results of spectra decomposed with various methods and tools: a) the Cromwell package b) the PrepMS tool c) the MassSpec Wavelet tool d) the PROcess package e) the mspeaks function (Matlab).

Single peaks are, in fact, modelled with single Gaussians. The appropriate choice of distribution parameters allows the representation of peak shapes and measurement errors. It is also easy to write the model. It is worth paying attention to the fact that single Gaussians might be used only in the case of perfectly-separated peaks. In practice, the analysis of the real spectra is done using mixtures of Gaussian distributions. Using a mixture of Gaussian distributions instead of single Gaussian distributions additionally takes account of interactions between closely-located peaks. Mass spectra reflect a number of processes occurring in an organism. Those processes are usually correlated with each other. They have their representation in the characterising spectra, especially in the lack of separability among its particular peaks. This fact needs to be considered during the analysis. The application of mixture models allows the considering of dependences between spectral peaks. It also facilitates the modelling of overlapped measuring errors placed in adjacent regions of the spectrum. Separate-peak identification could be a case of the incorrect assessment of the individual Gaussians variances, because it is not possible to completely separate them. Mixture modelling makes it possible to detect all peaks simultaneously and correct measurement inaccuracies. However, mixture model parameter solving is a complicated task that needs the determination of many properties like the number of components, the type of stop criterion or calculation accuracy.

3. Data classification

Preprocessing steps and decomposition are the first steps in the analysis. The second is classification, which might be used in the process of significant peak determination. Classification allows the search for the distinction between ill and healthy patients. It is also possible to look for the stage of disease progression or to check reactions (positive or negative) to medical treatment.

Classification of mass spectra collection is an essential but also difficult task, because of the specificity of the data. The most common classification tasks are based on the supervised learning. It usually consists of categorising data into two groups (for example ill and healthy). There are also attempts to classify data into three or more groups. Such classification tasks are, however, more complicated and they are not included in this chapter.

Classified objects are usually represented by vectors of observed, measured or calculated features. Supervised learning classification assumes that the unknown function Φ is to be assigned to each object of population O as a label of one class. The classification process is based on the learning set U which is a subset of the whole data set O. Each element o_i of the learning set is composed of the object representation and a class label. This object representation is an observation vector of the features. The whole set is divided into c separated subsets and one-subset observations are numbered among one of the c classes. Such supervised learning is widely used in biomedical applications.

3.1 Classifiers construction

·The construction of classifiers is based on several rules. Multiple different classifiers might be constructed on the basis of one single learning set. The ideal situation would be to choose the proper classifier on the basis of the number of misclassifications of the new, random observation. However, in reality bad classification probabilities are unknown. They might be estimated from a validation probe, which is a random sample, independent of the learning probe, where objects' belonging to classes are unknown. The misclassification probability of a specific classifier is estimated with mistakes done by the classifier on the validation probe. Classifier evaluation should be done using observations independent of those from the learning probe. In other cases the classifier will be biased.

The ultimate classifier evaluation is done with a test probe. It needs to be independent of other probes and it needs to have information about objects' membership of classes. If only one classifier is to be tested or basis size of the set is small, the validation probe might be omitted. In practice, the usually-chosen proportion is the division into 50% on the learning probe and 25% each for the validation and test probes (Cwik & Koronacki, 2008). However, in practice, the division depends on the specificity of the data set.

The classifier makes the decision about the belonging to classes on the basis of the learning probe. However, the trained classifier will need to operate on large datasets. These datasets are larger than sets used for classifier training. It makes non-zero the probability of a wrong decision (Stapor, 2005). The classifier is used for data other than those for which it was constructed. That is why the classifier quality depends on its generalisation ability. In practice it means that the learning properties need to be representative of all the population. On the other hand, nonessential properties should be omitted, because they only constitute features of the specific learning set.

The most popular measures of classification quality are classification accuracy (a proportion of correctly-classified sets) and error rate (a proportion of misclassified sets). Important rates are also TP (True Positives) – the number of correctly-classified positive sets, TN (True

Negatives) – the number of correctly-classified negative sets, FP (False Positives) – the number of incorrectly-classified positive sets, FN (False Negatives) – the number of incorrectly-classified negative sets.

Among useful measures one can also find sensitivity and specificity. This sensitivity is defined as a proportion of truly positive and false negative results (eq. 6). It is interpreted as ability of a classifier to identify the phenomenon if it really exists.

$$sensitivity = \frac{TP}{FN + TP} \qquad (6)$$

On the other hand the specificity is a proportion of truly negative results and the sum of truly negative and truly positive results (eq. 7). The specificity is interpreted as the ability to reject truly false results.

$$specificity = \frac{TN}{TN + FP} \qquad (7)$$

Sensitivity and specificity are opposed values – an increase in the one causes a decrease in the other.

The significant tool characterising a classifier's features is the receiver-operating-characteristic curve – known as the ROC curve. It is a chart of dependency between values: 1-specificity and sensitivity. Such a curve is created for a specific structure of the classifier (specified type, parameters, number of input features). The total error of the classifier remains unchanged. However, its division into values FP and FN is changed, because the ROC curve examines the proportion between FP and FN. In the case of the random division of objects, the ROC curve takes the shape of a curve going from the bottom left to the upper right corner. The better the classification results are, the more concave the curve is. The ideal situation will make the ROC curve go through the upper left corner of the chart.

An important factor in the classifier's quality is the curve under the ROC curve, the so-called AUC. The closer to the value 1 AUC is, the better are the classification results. An example of ROC is presented in Fig 6.

3.2 Dealing with high dimensionality

Mass spectrometry data are characterised by high dimensionality. The number of observations is significantly lower than the number of features. Each patient has a few thousand data points or even more, whereas a typical dataset contains dozens or hundreds of spectra. Typical classification and data mining techniques are designed to handle low-dimensional data, such as sales or economic indicators. Low-dimensional datasets contain many observations and just only a few, usually uncorrelated, features. Such data might be analysed using any type of method, including graphical interpretation and unsupervised learning. Dealing with high-dimensional data is much more difficult. The main problem is the correlation of features which always occur in high-dimensional data. In fact, to obtain statistical significance the number of observations should grow exponentially with the dimensionality. The existence of dependent features prevents or hinders the classification

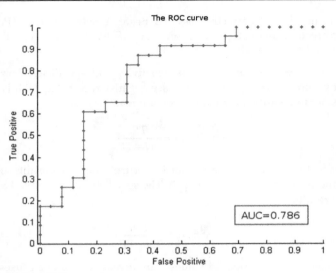

Fig. 6. Example of the ROC curve.

using typical, widely-known methods. Moreover, a large number of correlated features has a bad influence on the quality of the classification. This makes analysis difficult and diversification is hard to obtain (Stapor, 2005). A large number of features causes also large number of classifier parameters. It increases its complexity and susceptibility to over-learning and decreases its flexibility. The existence of the curse of dimensionality (Mao et al., 2000) proves that the complexity of the classifier has an impact on the classification quality. The more complex the classifier is, the higher should be the proportion between the number of observations and the number of features (Stapor, 2005). That is why high-dimensional data must be properly processed, including the application of dimension-reduction techniques. This task determines the success of the classification because of specificity of mass spectral data.

Another problem of dealing with bio-medical data is signal strength. A typical signal of mass spectrometry data carries information concerning the functions of the whole organism. Moreover, the development of medical, diagnostic and prevention programmes gives results for significantly less patients diagnosed with late-stage diseases. For example, cancer diseases are usually diagnosed at the first or second clinical level. Such signals are difficult to identify and to extract among the many different signals of the organism. Blood, serum or urine contain proteins responsible for the range of typical, vital functions of the body. One needs to notice that those proteins are much stronger than the signals of diseases.

One of the most frequently-used classifiers for mass spectrometry data is the Support Vectors Machines (SVM) proposed by V.N. Vapnik (Vapnik et al., 1992; Vapnik, 1995; Vapnik, 1998). The idea of this method is a classification using an appropriately-designated discriminant hyperplane. Searching for such a hyperplane is performed by the Mercer theorem and the optimisation of the quadratic objective function, with linear restrictions. The SVM idea is based on searching for two parallel hyperplanes. If classification groups are linearly separated, those hyperplanes should delimit the widest possible area which contain no elements of the probe. The hyperplanes need to be based on so-called support vectors. If learning sub-sets are not linearly separated, a penalty is introduced. The best separation result is obtained for a higher dimensional space.

The SVM rule is presented in Eq. 8.

$$f(x) = \text{sgn}(\sum_{sup.\ vect.} y_i \alpha_i^0 (x_i x) + b^0) \tag{8}$$

where α are Lagrange's coefficients and b is a constant value. For inseparable classes the additional restrictions take the form of Eq. 9.

$$x_i w + b \geq 1 - \xi_i, y_i = 1$$
$$x_i w + b \geq -1 + \xi_i, y_i = -1 \tag{9}$$

where ξ_i is a constant value $\xi_i \geq 0$

Classifiers used in bioinformatics applications are solved with use of kernel functions. Such a construction enables one to obtain non-linear shapes of discriminant hyperplanes. One of the most popular kernel functions is the radial kernel (Eq. 10).

$$f(x) = \text{sgn}(\sum_{sup.\ vect.} y_i \alpha_i^0 K(x_i x) + b^0) \tag{10}$$

Before the main classification of mass spectrometry data, dimension reduction needs to be performed. Input data-sets for classification usually contain several hundreds or even thousands of features. From the statistical point of view, using such a number of features is unreasonable. Reduction might be carried out in two-stages. The first is spectrum decomposition, which reduces dimensionality from thousands of features to hundreds. The second step is applying feature reduction or selection techniques.

The first step in dimension reduction is based on applying the decomposition results. These results are used as a Gaussian mask, which is put on every single spectrum of the data set. This gives new values consisting of all spectra. Dimensions of mass spectrometry data decrease to the value of the GMM components number. The resultant matrix obtained after these steps is $n \times k$, where n denoted the number of spectra and k the number of components. The resultant matrix was the input data to the further dimension reduction and classification.

There are many reduction and selection techniques available. They attempt to find the smallest data sub-set chosen with defined criteria among the whole data set. Too large a number of features has an adverse impact on the classification results. A large number of features causes an increase in computational complexity and lengthen calculation time. There are two types of dimension reduction methods:

- feature extraction – data are subjected to certain transformation – a new data set is obtained

• feature selection – a subset of the most optimal data is chosen.

One of commonly-known features extraction methods is the Partial Least Squares (PLS) method (Barnhill et al., 2002). The method also facilitates classification. Feature selection in the PLS method is performed with use of both X and Y data, so it considers the whole structure of the learning set. The idea of the PLS method is to find latent vectors. Using latent vectors allows simultaneous analysis and the decomposition of X and Y, including a covariance between X and Y. Such an approach makes PLS a special case of Principal Component Analysis (PCA) (Mao et al., 2000). The original version of PLS is a regression method dealing with continuous values. Classification of mass spectrometry data usually consists of assigning data to one of two groups. So, the matrix of dependent features (Y) is composed of only two values. It is possible to directly apply PLS to mass spectrometry or microarray data. However, it is better to use one of the few PLS modifications dedicated to binary classification. The original PLS classification components are a linear combination of predictor variables. Weights, however, are a nonlinear combination of predictor and response variables (Nguyen & Rockeb, 2004). There are approaches (Liu & Rayens, 2007; Boulesteix & Strimmer, 2006; Fort & Lambert-Lacroix, 2005; Nguyen & Rockeb, 2004; Man et al., 2004; Huang et al., 2005) applying the original PLS to categorical, binary responses. However, research confirms that it is better to use PLS procedures adjusted to binary responses (Nguyen & Rockeb, 2002). One can use a hybrid-PLS method based on singular-value decomposition. Another approach is the hybrid-PLS method based on logistic regression predictors, where the PLS components are calculated as weighted averages of the original predictor/explanatory variables. Also, weights are dependent on sample predictor variances and the partial correlation coefficient (Garthwaite, 1994; Nguyen & Rockeb, 2004). PLS is also used in conjunction with Linear Discriminant Analysis (LDA) (Boulesteix & Strimmer, 2006; Boulesteix, 2004; Liu & Rayens, 2007). Fort and Lambert-Lacroix (Fort & Lambert-Lacroix, 2005) proposed a combination of the PLS and Ridge penalty.

Among the most popular features selection method one can find the SVM-RFE and traditional T test. The SVM-RFE (Support Vector Machine Recursive Feature Elimination) (Wold, 1996) method is a features-selection method. Features selection is performed with the propagation-backward method. The procedure starts with a full range of input features and features are successively removed. Only one feature is removed at a time. As a range criterion SVM weights coefficients are used. Therefore the SVM-RFE method is closely related to the SVM classification. The T test is a very common technique of feature selection. The most significant features are chosen according the T test. For each feature a T-test range is calculated. This statistics treat all features as independent and this assumption is usually not met. However, the T test is successfully used for protein data classification.

3.3 Learning the classifier

After applying dimension reduction, supervised classification is preformed with the SVM method. Our results (Plechawska-Wójcik, 2011) show that the best results can be obtained using linear SVM and SVM with the Gaussian Radial Basis Function kernel. However, before the learning process, proper classification parameters need to be estimated. Such an estimation is usually performed experimentally, for example using the Multiple Random Validation method.

Tests of classification and reduction performance need to be done for different values of the SVM parameters and the number of selected features. To find the most accurate values, the dataset must be divided into testing and learning subsets. Classification calculations need to be repeated several hundred times. The classification analysis should be performed separately for all used dimension reduction techniques. Each of them can have a different number of obtained features. Besides the total error, False Negatives and False Positives should be also checked.

The SVM parameters are the value of box constraints (C) for the soft margin and the scaling factor (sigma). The results of multiple repetitions of SVM for different sigma values are presented in Fig. 7. The classification was done with SVM classifier with a radial kernel. All calculations were done in the Matlab environment.

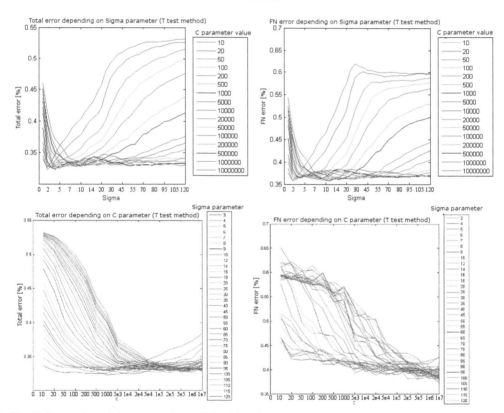

Fig. 7. Examples of the estimation of classification parameters.

If parameters are already known, there is a necessity to find the optimal number of features. For example, if there is a 50-element learning-data set, number of features shouldn't be larger than 10. The results for all three types of dimension-reduction techniques are presented in Fig. 8. The middle line is the obtained ratio and the upper and lower denotes the confidence interval. Similar results are obtained for the FN and FP values.

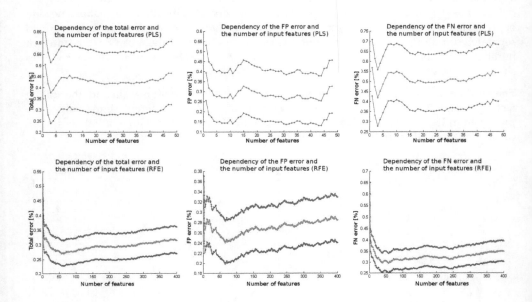

Fig. 8. Examples of the estimation of the features number.

4. The biological interpretation of mass spectrometry data

Another important issue in mass spectrometry data analysis is the supporting of biological interpretation. The ability to check the details of those components is of great importance to biologists. Biological interpretation tries to determine peptides and proteins on the basis of the m/z values list. After this identification further analysis can be performed. The application gives characteristics of found peptides and proteins. It is also able to find characteristics of genes coding the proteins and to give access to genes paths. The biological context module is integrated with four biological databases available online.

At level0 the user is able to load data and give detailed search criteria. These criteria include accuracy, species, the MS platform, and the possibility of double and triple charges. Searching is based on M/Z values, which are transferred from classification module.

Level1 is based on the EPO-KB (Empirical Proteomic Ontology Knowledge Base) database (Lustgarten et al., 2008; Lustgarten et al., 2009). The names of proteins and peptides are found on the basis of given M/Z values with a specified percentage tolerance. The user can also see the original results in the EPO-KB service.

Level2 is a protein level and data presented here are obtained from an UniProt (Jain et al., 2009) database. The displayed results contain detailed information about proteins, such as entry name, status of reviewing process, organism, gene names and identifiers, features and GO annotations. It is also possible to see the original results returned by the database.

Level3 is a genes level and it gives information about genes coding a particular protein chosen at a previous level2. Presented data are based on NCBI service (Wheeler, 2009). Searching is based on a gene identifier and it returns precise information about a particular gene, its role, status, lineage and related data. Level4 is based on gene pathways data. It is integrated with the KEGG database (Kyoto Encyclopedia of Genes and Genomes) (Kanehisa, 2008). Level 4 gives details about gene pathways, structures, sequences, and references to other databases.

An example of biological results obtained at the level of proteins is presented in Fig. 10. More results of the analysis performed on real data are presented in (Plechawska-Wojcik, 2011a).

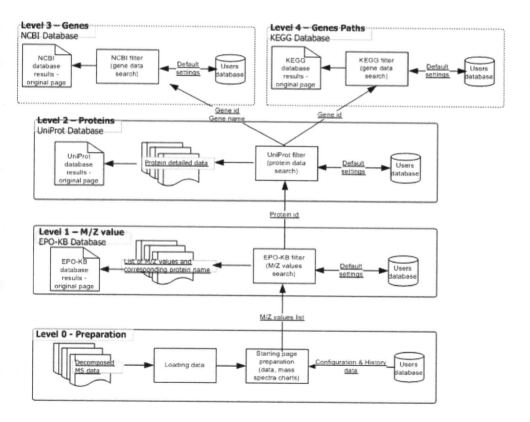

Fig. 9. Schema of a biological-interpretation module.

Accesion	EntryName	Status	ProteinNames	GeneNames	Organism	Length	Szczegóły
P02656	APOC3_HUMAN	reviewed	Apolipoprotein C-III (Apo-CIII) (ApoC-III) (Apolipoprotein C3)	APOC3	Homo sapiens (Human)	99	Więcej
P02647	APOA1_HUMAN	reviewed	Apolipoprotein A-I (Apo-AI) (ApoA-I) (Apolipoprotein A1) [Cleaved into: Apolipoprotein A-I(1-242)]	APOA1	Homo sapiens (Human)	267	Więcej
P06727	APOA4_HUMAN	reviewed	Apolipoprotein A-IV (Apo-AIV) (ApoA-IV) (Apolipoprotein A4)	APOA4	Homo sapiens (Human)	396	Więcej
A3KPE2	A3KPE2_HUMAN	unreviewed	Apolipoprotein C-III (Apolipoprotein C-III variant 2) (Apolipoprotein C-III variant 3) (Apolipoprotein C-III, isoform CRA_a)	APOC3 hCG_41334	Homo sapiens (Human)	99	Więcej
Q6Q788	APOA5_HUMAN	reviewed	Apolipoprotein A-V (Apo-AV) (ApoA-V) (Apolipoprotein A5) (Regeneration-associated protein 3)	APOA5 RAP3 UNQ411/PRO773	Homo sapiens (Human)	366	Więcej
B0YIW2	B0YIW2_HUMAN	unreviewed	Apolipoprotein C-III variant 1	APOC3	Homo sapiens (Human)	117	Więcej

Fig. 10. An example of biological analysis at the protein level.

5. Conclusion

The presented project is a comprehensive bioinformatics approach enabling spectra pre-processing and analysing. The use of the Gaussian Mixture Model decomposition facilitates particular work with different types of spectra, especially complex, containing overlapped peaks. Before the analysis, one needs to choose the proper settings adjusted to the specificity of data. It is a condition of successful analysis. To minimise the risk of improper parameters selection, a parameters test should be performed.

All elements of the mass spectrometry data analysis process are closely related. Each performed operation has an influence on the further quality of results. Preprocessing analysis is especially essential for the final results. That is why it is necessary to perform it in the correct order and using the proper parameter set. Some operations, however, are performed optionally and are chosen by the user.

We found the peak-detection method based on Gaussian Mixture Models slower than common spectra analysis techniques based on local maxima and minima. However, it can deal with different kinds of data including spectra with overlapped peaks.

Mixture model parameters are estimated using the Expectation-Maximisation algorithm with appropriately-selected parameters. It enables to obtain reproducible, reliable results. The decomposition carried out in this way allows the detection of peaks which can be subjected to further analysis, like protein and peptide identification, biomarker detection and the allocation of the tested sample to one of target groups.

Classification allows the initial indication of the power of the predictive model and the functional analysis of detected peaks. It is, however, a difficult task, due to the high dimensionality and feature correlation. Many thousands of features and tens of objects require two-step dimensionality reduction. The first one is based on the Gaussian mask, imposed on all spectra of the dataset. The second is the separation of the most informative features, conducted by the dimensionality-reduction techniques. Due to the high correlation degree, the classification should be based on features. Before the classification procedure the classifier parameters need to be specified.

The last step of the analysis is the biological interpretation. Biological databases integration facilitates the verification of the results. This test is important because of the possible False Discovery Rate obtained during the raw spectra analysis and classification. Such verification gives the possibility to verify the analysis from another angle. Biological analysis based on several external databases gives reliable functional analysis. Source databases are updated frequently. This ensures reliable, actual results.

6. Acknowledgment

The author is grateful to Prof. Joanna Polańska for inspiration, many invaluable suggestions and assistance in the preparation of this paper.

7. References

Akaike, H. (1974). A new look at the statistical model identification. *IEEE Transactions on Automatic Control*, 9, pp. 716–723.

Banfield, J. & Raftery, A. (1993). Model-based gaussian and non-gaussian clustering. *Biometrics*, 49, p.803–821.

Barnhill, S.; Vapnik, V.; Guyon, I. & Weston, J. (2002). Gene selection for cancer classification using support vector machines. *Machine Learning*, 46, pp. 389–422.

Boulesteix, A. (2004). PLS dimension reduction for classification with high-dimensional microarray data. *StatAppl GenetMol Biol*, 3, pp. 33.

Boulesteix, A. & Strimmer, K. (2006). Partial least squares: a versatile tool for the analysis of high-dimensionalgenomic data. *Briefings In Bioinformatics*, 8(1), pp. 32-44.

Bozdogan, H. (1990). On the information-based measure of covariance complexity and its application to the evaluation of multivariate linear models. *Communications in Statictics, Theory and Methods*, 19, p. 221–278.

Bozdogan, H. (1993) Choosing the number of component clusters in the mixture-model using a new informational complexity criterion of the inverse-fisher informational matrix. *Springer-Verlag*,Heidelberg, 19, pp. 40–54.

Celeux G. & Soromenho G. (1996). An entropy criterion for assessing the number of clusters in a mixture model. *Classification Journal*, 13, pp. 195–212.

Coombes, K.; Baggerly, K. & Morris, J. (2007). Pre-processing mass spectrometry data. *Fundamentals of Data Mining in Genomics and Proteomics*, in : W. Dubitzky, M. Granzow, and D. Berrar, (Eds.), pp. 79-99, Kluwer, Boston.

Cwik, J. & Koronacki, J. (2008). *Statisitical learining systems*. Akademicka Oficyna Wydawnicza Exit Warszawa, pp. 239-245.

Dempster, A.P.; Laird, N.M. & Rubin D.B. (1977). Maximum likelihood from incomplete data via the em algorithm. *J. R. Stat. Soc.*, 39,1:1 — 38.

Du, P.; Kibbe, W. & Lin S. (2006). Improved peak detection in mass spectrum by incorporating continuous wavelet transform-based pattern matching. *Bioinformatics*, Vol. 22 no. 17 2006, 2059-2065.

Eidhammer, I.; Flikka, K.; Martens L. & Mikalsen S. (2007). *Computational methods for mass spectrometry proteomics*, John Wiley and sons.

Everitt B.S. & Hand D.J. (1981). *Finite Mixture Distributions*, Chapman and Hall, New York.

Fort, G. & Lambert-Lacroix, S. (2005). Classification using partial least squares with penalized logistic regression. *Bioinformatics*, 21(7), pp. 1104–1111.

Fung, E.T. & Enderwick C. (2002) ProteinChip clinical proteomics: computational challenges and solutions, *Biotechniques*, Suppl., 32, pp. 34-41.

Garthwaite, P.H. (1994). An interpretation of partial least squares. *J. Amer. Statist. Assoc.*, 89, pp. 122–127.

Guindani, M.; Do, K.; Mueller, P. & Morris, J. (2006). Bayesian Mixture Models for Gene Expression and Protein Profiles. *Bayesian Inference for Gene Expression and Proteomics*. KA Do, P Mueller, M Vannucci (Eds.) New York: Cambridge University Press, pp. 238-253.

Huang, X.; Pan, W.; Grindle, S.; et al. (2005). A comparative study of discriminating human heart failure etiology using gene expression profiles. *BMC Bioinformatics*, 6, pp. 205.

Jain, E.; Bairoch, A.; Duvaud, S.; Phan, I.; Redaschi, N.; Suzek, B.E.; Martin, M.J.; McGarvey, P. & Gasteiger E. (2009). Infrastructure for the life sciences: design and implementation of the UniProt website. *BMC Bioinformatics* 10, pp. 136.

Kanehisa, M.; Araki, M.; Goto, S.; Hattori, M.; Hirakawa, M.; Itoh, M.; Katayama, T.; Kawashima, S.; Okuda, S.; Tokimatsu, T. & Yamanishi, Y. (2008). KEGG for linking genomes to life and the environment. *Nucleic Acids Res.*, 36, D480-D484.

Liu, Y. & Rayens, W. (2007). PLS and dimension reduction for classification. *Computational Statistics*, 22, pp. 189–208.

Lustgarten, J.L.; et al. (2008). EPO-KB: a searchable knowledge base of biomarker to protein links. *Bioinformatics*, 24(11), pp. 1418-1419.

Lustgarten, J.L.; et al. (2009). Knowledge-based variable selection for learning rules from proteomic data. *Bioinformatics*, 10(Suppl 9), S16.

Man, M.Z.; Dyson G.; Johnson K., et al. (2004). Evaluating methods for classifying expression data. *J Biopharm Stat*, 14, 1065–84.

Mantini, D.; Petrucci, F., Del Boccio, P.; Pieragostino, D.; Di Nicola, M.; Lugaresi, A.; Federici, G.; Sacchetta, P.; Di Ilio, C. & URBANI A. (2008). Independent component analysis for the extraction of reliable protein signal profiles from MALDI-TOF mass spectra, *Bioinformatics*, 24, 63-70.

Mantini, D.; Petrucci, F.; Pieragostino, D.; Del Boccio, P.; Di Nicola, M.; Di Ilio, C.; Federici, G.; Sacchetta, P.; Comani, S. & URBANI A. (2007) LIMPIC: a computational method for the separation of protein signals from noise, *BMC Bioinformatics*, 8, 101.

Mao, J.; Jain, A.K. & Duin, R.P.W. (2000). Statistical pattern recognition: a review. *IEEE Trans.* PAMI, 22(1): pp. 4–37.

Morris, J.; Coombes, K.; Kooman, J.; Baggerly, K. & Kobayashi, R. (2005) Feature extraction and quantification for mass spectrometry data in biomedical applications using the mean spectrum. *Bioinformatics*, 21(9), pp. 1764-1775.

Nguyen, D. & Rocke D. Tumor classification by partial least squares using microarray gene expression data. *Bioinformatics*, 18, pp. 39–50.

Nguyen, D. & Rockeb, D. (2004). On partial least squares dimension reduction for microarray-based classification: a simulation study. *Computational Statistics & Data Analysis*, 46, pp. 407–425.

Plechawska, M. (2008a). Comparing and similarity determining of Gaussian distributions mixtures. *Polish Journal of Environmental Studies*, Vol.17, No. 3B, Hard Olsztyn, pp. 341-346.

Plechawska, M. (2008b). Using mixtures of Gaussian distributions for proteomic spectra analysis, *International Doctoral Workshops, OWD 2008 Proceedings*, pp. 531-536.

Polanska, J.; Plechawska, M.; Pietrowska, M. & Marczak, L. (2011). Gaussian Mixture decomposition in the analysis of MALDI-ToF spectra. *Expert Systems*, doi: 10.1111/j.1468-0394. 2011. 00582.x, 2011.

Plechawska-Wójcik M. (2011a). Biological interpretation of the most informative peaks in the task of mass spectrometry data classification. *Studia Informatica. Zeszyty Naukowe Politechniki Śląskiej, seria INFORMATYKA*. Vol.32, 2A (96). Wydawnictwo Politechniki Śląskiej, 2011, pp. 213-228.

Plechawska-Wójcik M. (2011b). Comprehensive analysis of mass spectrometry data – a case study. *Contemporary Economics*. Univeristy of Finanse and Management in Warsaw.

Randolph, T.; Mithcell, B.; Mclerran, D.; Lampe, P. & Feng Z. (2005). Quantifying peptide signal in MALDI-TOF mass spectrometry data. *Molecular & cellular proteomics, MCP*, 4 (12), pp. 1990-9.

Schwarz, G. (1978). Estimating the dimension of a model. *Annals of Statistics*, 6, p. 461–464.

Stapor, K. (2005). *Automatic objects classification*. Akademicka Oficyna Wydawnicza Exit Warszawa, pp. 35-52.

Tibshirani, R.; Hastiey, T.; Narasimhanz, B.; Soltys, S.; Shi, G.; Koong A. & Le, Q.T. (2004) Sample classification from protein mass spectrometry, by 'peak probability contrasts'. *Bioinformatics*, 20, pp. 3034 - 3044.

Vapnik, V.; Boster, B. & Guyon, I. (1992). A training algorithm for optimal margin classifiers. *Fifth Annual Workshop on Computational Learning Theory*, pp. 114–152.

Vapnik, V. (1995). *The Nature of Statistical Learning Theory*. Springer.

Vapnik, V. (1998). *Statistical Learning Theory*. Wiley.

Wheeler DL et al. (2009). Database resources of the National Center for Biotechnology Information. *Nuc. Acids Res.*, 37, D5-D15.

Windham, M.P. & Cutler A. (1993). Information ratios for validating cluster analyses. *Journal of the American Statistical Association*, 87:1188–1192.

Wold, H. (1996). Estimation of principal components and related models by iterative least squares. Multivariate Analysis, *Academic Press*, New York, pp. 391-420.

Yasui, Y.; Pepe, M.; Thompson, M.L.; Adam, B.L.; Wright, Y. Qu.; Potter, J.D.; Winget, M.; Thornquist M. & Feng Z. (2003). A data-analytic strategy for protein biomarker discovery: profiling of highdimensional proteomic data for cancer detection. *Biostatistics*, 4, pp. 449-463.

Zhang, S.Q.; Zhou, X.; Wang, H.; Suffredini, A.; Gonzales, D.; Ching, W.K.; Ng, M. & Wong
    S. (2007). Peak detection with chemical noise removal using Short-Time FFT for
    a kind of MALDI Data, *Proceedings of OSB 2007*, Lecture Notes in Operations
    Research, 7, pp. 222-231.

4

Aligning Biomedical Terminologies in French: Towards Semantic Interoperability in Medical Applications

Tayeb Merabti[1], Lina F. Soualmia[1,2], Julien Grosjean[1],
Michel Joubert[3] and Stefan J. Darmoni[1]
[1]CISMeF, Rouen University Hospital, Normandy & TIBS, LITIS EA 4108,
Institute of Biomedical Research, Rouen
[2]LIM & Bio EA 3969, Paris XIII University, Sorbonne Paris Cité, Bobigny
[3]LERTIM EA 3283, Faculty of Medicine, Marseilles
France

1. Introduction

In health, there exist practically as many different terminologies, controlled vocabularies, thesauri and classification systems as there are fields of application. In fact, terminologies play important roles in clinical data capture, annotation, reporting, information integration, indexing and retrieval. These knowledge sources have mostly different formats and purposes. For example, among many other knowledge sources, the Systematized NOmenclature of MEDicine International (SNOMED Int) is used for clinical coding, the French CCAM for procedures, the 10th revision of the International Classification of Diseases (ICD10) and the Anatomical Therapeutic Chemical (ATC) Classification for drugs are used for epidemiological and medico-economic purposes and the Medical Subject Headings (MeSH) thesaurus for indexing bibliographic databases. Given the great number of terminologies, existing tools, such as search engines, coding systems or decision support systems, are limited in dealing with "syntactic" and "semantic" divergences in spite of their great storage capacity and quick processing of data. Faced with this reality and the increasing need to allow cooperation with/between the various health actors and their related health information systems, it appears necessary to link and connect these terminologies to make them "interoperable". The objective is to allow the different actors to speak the same language while using different representations of the same things. As it is essential to render these terminologies "interoperable", this involves establishing a joint semantic repository to allow effective interaction with a minimum loss of meaning. This semantic interoperability requires a shared model, i.e. a common representation of terms and concepts, whatever the original terminology or repository is but it also requires the development of methods to allow connection between equivalent terms or relations from each terminology.

Various studies have investigated the implementation of platforms to achieve interoperability between health terminologies. The Unified Medical Language System (UMLS), developed by the US National Library of Medicine since 1986 (Lindberg et al., 1993), is one such project.

Currently, it is considered as the largest existing metathesaurus. However, the UMLS does not make semantically integrated terminology interoperable but rather provides rich health knowledge sources that can potentially be used towards mapping or connection identification. Other studies were interested in the issue of providing terminology servers in the health domain (Chute et al., 1999; Rector et al., 1997). The use of multiple terminologies is recommended to increase the number of lexical and graphical forms of a biomedical term recognized by a search engine. For this reason, in France, since 2005, the Catalog and Index of Health Resources in French (CISMeF) has evolved from a mono-terminology approach using MeSH main headings and subheadings to a multiple terminologies paradigm using, in addition to the MeSH thesaurus, several vocabularies and classifications that deal with various aspects of health.The overall CISMeF Information System (CISMeF_IS), includes multiple-terminologies indexing (Pereira et al., 2008), multi-terminology information retrieval (Sakji et al., 2009; Soualmia et al., 2011) and integrates of several terminologies (n=32) in the CISMeF terminology database. The CISMeF team has created a Health Multi-Terminology Portal (HMTP) largely inspired by the most recent advances in semantic web technologies (Darmoni et al., 2009a). Besides platforms, terminology servers and other computer systems for semantic interoperability, there are significant challenges in developing automated and semi-automated approaches for identifying direct and indirect relations between terms i.e. alignments. Aligning different terminologies by determining relations is a hard task regardless of the research field, whether in Information Science (Zeng & Chan, 2004), matching database schemas (Doan et al., 2004) or aligning ontologies (Euzenat & Shvaiko, 2007). In addition to heterogeneity formats, two problems complicate the alignments between terminologies. Firstly, the informal processing of relations in the terminology which makes several definitions ambiguous (Sarker et al., 2003). Unfortunately, this problem remains difficult to solve because it requires changes in the logical construction of each original terminology: hierarchical relationships, synonymy relations or related relations. The second problem consists in making these approaches automatic. In fact, most of the existing approaches to link terminologies are manual and very time consuming. For example, the manual mapping between ATC and the MeSH thesaurus took more than 6 men.months. Obviously, it is not possible for a team such as CISMeF (n=20) or another team of the same scale to manually produce at least 190 mappings between 32 terminologies$\frac{N(N-1)}{2}$. In this chapter, we aim primarily to contribute to the second problem related to the automation of mapping approaches to identify relations between terminologies. The remainder of the chapter is organized as follows: in section 2 we start by a panel of several biomedical terminologies (including classifications, controlled vocabularies, taxonomies, . . .etc).

Some projects (UMLS and the HMTP) for integrating medical terminologies and ontologies are described in the section 3. The section 4 is devoted to background on terminology and on ontology alignments methods, mainly semantic and syntactic ones. The methods we propose are developed in the section 5. Alignments of specific terminologies are presented in the section 6 and the section 7 displays the global results we have obtained. The section 8 gives several uses of the alignments through the HMTP, mainly for information retrieval and automatic translation. Finally some related work and discuss the results we have obtained and conclude this study in sections 9 and 10.

2. Panel of biomedical terminologies and their use

2.1 Terminology definition

A terminological system links together concepts of a domain and gives their associated terms, and sometimes their definition and code. It might take the designation of *terminology, thesausrus, controlled vocabulary, nomenclature, classification, taxonomy* or *ontology*. In (Roche, 2005), terminology was defined as a set of words. A more precise definition of terminology was given in (Lefevre, 2000): "Terminologies are a list of terms of one area or a topic representing concepts or notions most frequently used or most characteristic". Thereby, the content and the structure of a terminology depend on the function for which this terminology will be used.

A terminology in which the terms are for example organized alphabetically and in which the concepts may be designed with one or several synonyms is a *thesaurus*. When the terms are associated to definitions, it constitutes a *controlled vocabulary*. A *nomenclature* is a terminology in which the terms are composed according to pre-existing rules. When hierarchical relations are introduced between concepts, it is a classification. A *classification* is the exhaustive organization of the concepts of a domain into classes, according to their distinctive characteristics. The classes are mutually exclusive and organized hierarchically from the most generic to the most specific. In classifications, one can find classes denoted "No Otherwise Specified" which gather terms that cannot be classified elsewhere. A *taxonomy* is a classification in which the classes have only hierarchical relations of generic type.

In medical terminologies, specific terms are used to specify concepts of the domain. Relations can also exist between terms. For example, generalization and specialization relations (is-a) exist in several terminologies to rank terms from the more general to the more specific, and partitive ones (part-of) designs which term designates a part-of another one. In terminologies, concepts can be designated by several different terms. A Preferred Term (PT) is the term describing a unique medical concept in terminology. The PT is defined as less ambiguous, more specific and self-descriptive as possible. As a continuum with terminology, an ontology is a "formal, explicit specification of a shared conceptualization for a domain of interest" (Gruber, 1993). Usually, an ontology is organized by concepts and identifies all possible inter-relations. Ontologies are used to facilitate communication among domain experts and between domain experts and knowledge-based systems. This is done to reflect the expert view of a specific domain. The difference with terminology, is mainly in knowledge representation language, which is formal in the case of ontology.

2.2 The main medical terminologies

In this section we describe several terminologies. As explained in the introduction, each terminology is developed for a particular use. The following terminologies are the most known in the domain of health:

- the main thesaurus used for medical information is the Medical Subject Headings (MeSH®) (Nelson et al., 2001) maintained by the U.S. National Library of Medicine. It consists of a controlled vocabulary used for indexing the content of health documents and it is available in 41 languages, including 26,000 MeSH Descriptors, 83 MeSH Qualifiers and 200,000 MeSH Supplementary Concepts (MeSH SC) ;

- The Systematized Nomenclature Of MEDicine (SNOMED) International is used essentially to describe electronic health records (Côté et al., 1993), and is a standard for electronic health records (Cornet & de Keizer, 2008);
- Medical Dictionary for Regulatory Activities (MedDRA), for adverse effects (Brown et al., 1999);
- Logical Observation Identifiers Names and Codes (LOINC) (Cormont et al., 2011);
- International Union of Pure and Applied Chemistry (IUPAC) for chemical sciences[1];
- Various codes used for drugs and chemical compounds: CAS for chemistry, Brand Names and International Non-proprietary Names (INN) for drugs.

Several terminologies are developed and maintained by the World Health Organization (WHO):

- The International Classification of Diseases, 10th revision (ICD10)[2];
- The Adverse Reactions Terminology (WHO-ART), for adverse effects[3];
- The Anatomical Therapeutic Chemical Classification System (WHO-ATC)[4] for drugs;
- The International Classification for Patient Safety (WHO-ICPS)[5];
- International Classification of Functioning, Disability and Health(WHO-ICF)[6] for handicap.

Concerning diseases, the ORPHANET thesaurus is available in five languages (English, French, Spanish, Italian and Portuguese). It describes rare diseases, including related genes and symptoms (Aymé et al., 1998). The MEDLINEPlus thesaurus (Miller et al., 2000) is a thesaurus for lay people. More formal representations exist. For example :

- Foundational Model of Anatomy (FMA) (Noy et al., 2004; Rosse & Mejino, 2003) which describes anatomical entities.
- Human Phenotype Ontology (HPO) (Robinson & Mundlos, 2010)

In France, the Joint Classification of Medical Procedures (CCAM) (Rodrigues et al., 1997) and ICD10 are mandatory for epidemiological and medico-economic purposes for all private and public health care institutions. The International Classification of Primary Care, Second edition (ICPC2) [7] and French dictionary for outpatients (DRC)[8] are two classifications for family medicine and primary care respectively designed by the World Organization of National Colleges (WONCA), Academies, and Academic Associations of General Practitioners/Family Physicians) and the French Society of Family Medicine (SFMG)). Two French terminologies exist to describe medical devices: LPP[9] and CLADIMED[10]. LPP is

---

[1] http://www.iupac.org/
[2] http://www.who.int/classifications/icd/en/
[3] http://www.umc-products.com
[4] http://www.whocc.no/atcddd/
[5] http://www.who.int/patientsafety/implementation/taxonomy/
[6] http://www.who.int/classifications/icf/en/
[7] http://www.who.int/classifications/icd/adaptations/icpc2/
[8] http://www.sfmg.org/outils_sfmg/dictionnaire_des_resultats_de_consultation-drc/
[9] http://www.codage.ext.cnamts.fr/codif/tips/index_presntation.php?p_site=AMELI
[10] http://www.cladimed.com

the list of medical devices from the French National Health Insurance and CLADIMED is a five level classification for medical devices, based on the ATC classification approach (same families). Devices are classified according to their main use and validated indications.

Another original way to represent medical concepts is the use of a graphical language based on pictograms, icons and colors with compositional rules (Lamy et al., 2008). We have presented a few examples of existing terminologies and their use. Development of techniques to allow semantic interoperability between these knowledge sources of heterogeneous formats and contents. In the following section we describe projects developed in the US and in France that have proposed efficient ways to connect several terminologies of different use, languages and formats.

3. Integrating medical terminologies for interoperability

3.1 The Unified Medical Language System (UMLS) Project

The richest source of biomedical terminologies, thesauri, classifications is constituted by the Unified Medical Language System (UMLS) Metathesaurus (Lindberg et al., 1993) initiated by the U.S. NLM (National Library of Medicine) with the purpose of integrating information from a variety of sources. It is a way of overcoming two major barriers to efficient retrieval of machine-readable information: (i) the different expression of the same concepts in different machine-readable sources and by different people; (ii) the distribution of useful information between databases and systems. The purpose of UMLS is to facilitate the development of computer systems that use the biomedical knowledge to understand biomedicine and health data and information. To that end, the NLM distributes two types of resources for use by system developers and computing researchers:

- The UMLS Knowledge Sources (databases) integrates over 2 million names for some 900,000 concepts from over 154 biomedical vocabularies from 60 families of vocabularies, as well as 12 million relations between these concepts used in patient records, administrative data, full-text databases and expert systems (Bodenreider, 2004). There are three UMLS Knowledge Sources: the Metathesaurus, the Semantic Network and the SPECIALIST Lexicon.

- Associated software tools to assist developers in customizing or using the UMLS Knowledge Sources for particular purposes. Some of the tools included are for example MetamorphoSys (a tool for customization of the Metathesaurus), Lexical Variant Generator (LVG) for generation of lexical variants of concept names or MetaMap (for extraction of UMLS concepts from texts).

The UMLS Metathesaurus is a very large, multi-purpose, and multilingual vocabulary database that contains information about biomedical and health-related concepts, their various names, and the relationships between them. It is built from the electronic versions of many different thesauri, classifications, code sets, and lists of controlled terms used in patient care, health services billing, public health statistics, biomedical literature indexing and cataloging, and health services research. All the terminologies are under a common representation. The Metathesaurus creates concepts from the various sources and assigns each concept a Concept Unique Identifier (CUI). A CUI may refer to multiple terms from the individual terminologies. These concepts are labeled with Atomic Unique Identifiers (AUIs). For example, the AUI *Cold Temperature* [A15588749] from MeSH and the AUI *Low Temperature*

[A3292554] from SNOMEDCT are mapped to the CUI *Cold Temperature* [C0009264]. Ambiguity arises in the Metathesaurus when a term maps to more than one CUI. For example, the term *cold* maps to the CUIs *Cold Temperature* [C0009264], the *Common Cold* [C0009443], *Cold Sensation* [C0234192], *Chronic Obstructive Lung Disease* [C0024117], or *Colds homeopathic medication* [C1949981] the meaning of which is correct depending on the context in which the term is used. Concept Unique Identifiers CUIs in the Metathesaurus denote possible meanings that a term may have in the Metathesaurus. A CUI is expressed by specific attributes that define it such as its: preferred term, associated terms (synonyms), concept definition, related concepts. For example, the CUI C0009264 has the preferred term *Cold Temperature*. The definition of *Cold Temperature* [C0009264] is: Having less heat energy than the object against which it is compared; the absence of heat. Some of the terms associated with *Cold Temperature* [C0009264] are: *Cold Temperature, Low Temperature, Cold Thermal Agent* and *Cold*. There are two different types of relations that can exist between concepts, subsumption relations (is-a) such as parent/child, and other relations such as siblings. For example, the parent of *Cold Temperature* [C0009264] is *Temperature* [C0039476] and one of its siblings is *Hot Temperature* [C2350229].

Among the 154 biomedical vocabularies, the UMLS Metathesaurus includes only six (6) French terminologies: the MeSH, ICD10, SNOMED Int, WHO-ART, ICPC2 and MedDRA. Nevertheless, only four (4) terminologies are included with their French version in UMLS Metathesaurus (MeSH, WHO-ART, WHO-ICPC2 and MedDRA). However, several translations have already been added, such as MEDLINEPlus (Deléger et al., 2010) and partially LOINC and FMA (Merabti et al., 2011). The SPECIALIST Lexicon provides the lexical information of many biomedical terms. The information available for each word or term records includes syntactic, morphological and orthographic information. This lexical information is very useful for natural language processing systems, specifically for the SPECIALIST NLP (Natural Language Processing) System. However, the SPECIALIST Lexicon contains only English biomedical terms and general English terms and the associated NLP tools stands for English. The Semantic Network provides a categorization of Metathesaurus concepts into semantic types and relationships between semantic types. It provides a set of useful relationships between concepts represented in the Metathesaurus and a consistent categorization of all these concepts The current release of the Semantic Network contains 135 semantic types and 54 relationsh. A semantic type is a cluster of concepts that are meaningfully related in some way. For example, the semantic type of *Cold Temperature* is *Natural Phenomenon or Process*, whereas *Temperature* is assigned the semantic type *Quantitative Concept*. A concept may be assigned more than one semantic type. Nonetheless, the Metathesaurus does not allow interoperability between terminologies since it integrates the various terminologies as they stand without making any connection between the terms in the terminologies other than by linking equivalent terms to a single identifier in the Metathesaurus. For example the concept *Addison's disease* [C0001403] corresponds to :

3.2 Health Multi Terminology Portal (HMTP)

Since 2005, the Catalog and Index of Health Resources in French (CISMeF) evolved from a mono-terminology approach using the MeSH main headings and subheadings to a multiple terminologies paradigm using, in addition to the MeSH thesaurus, several vocabularies and classifications that deal with various aspects of health. The CISMeF team has created a Health Multi-Terminology Portal (HMTP) largely inspired by the most recent advances in

Addison's disease	[SNOMEDCT]	PT363732003
Addison's Disease	[MedlinePlus]	PT1233
Addison Disease	[MeSH]	D000224
Addison's disease	[SNOMED CT]	PT363732003
Addison's Disease	[MedlinePlus]	T1233
Addison Disease	[MeSH]	D000224
Bronzed disease	[SNOMED 1998]	Int DB-70620
Deficiency; corticorenal, primary	[ICPC2-ICD10 Thesaurus]	THU021575
Primary Adrenal Insufficiency	[MeSH]	D000224
Primary hypoadreanlism syndrome, Addison	[MedDRA]	10036696

web technologies (Darmoni et al., 2009b; Grosjean et al., 2011). The HMTP includes all the terminologies listed in section 2.2 and others related to drugs : the International Union of Pure and Applied Chemistry (IUPAC) for chemical sciences, various codes used for drugs and chemical compounds: CAS for chemistry, Brand Names and International Non-proprietary Names (INN) for drugs, CIS, UCD, and CIP for French drugs.

The HMTP includes also a CISMeF thesaurus (Douyère et al., 2004), which is an extension to the MeSH thesaurus, includes 130 metaterms (super-concepts to unify MeSH terms of the same medical discipline), 300 resource types (adaptation to the Internet of the publication types), over 200 predefined queries and the translation of 12,000 MeSH Scope Notes (8,000 manually and the rest semi-automatically). To fit all the terminologies into one global structure and allow semantic interoperability, a generic model compliant with the terminology ISO model was designed. It was established around the "Descriptor" which is the central concept of the terminologies (aka "keyword"). The HMTP is a "Terminological Portal" connected to generic model database to search terms among all the health terminologies available in French (or in English and translated into French) and to search it dynamically. The ultimate goal is to use this search via the HMTP in order to: (i) manually or automatically index resources in the CISMeF catalog; (ii) allow multi-terminology information retrieval (Darmoni et al., 2009b; Soualmia et al., 2011).

It can also be very useful in teaching or performing audits in terminology management. Currently, the HMTP allows users to access 32 terminologies and classifications. Some of those are included in the UMLS meta-thesaurus (n=9) but the majority are not (n=23) such as the ORPHANET thesaurus (Aymé et al., 1998), DRC (Ferru & Kandel, 2003), IUPAC[11]. Table 1 lists most of the terminologies included in the HMTP and table 2 displays the number of descriptors and relationships included.

4. Semantic integration through alignments

4.1 Methods for aligning terminologies and ontologies

Ontology alignment is the task of determining correspondences between concepts of different ontologies. A set of correspondences is also called an alignment (Euzenat & Shvaiko, 2007).

---

[11] IUPAC: http://www.iupac.org

Terminology	HMTP	UMLS
CCAM	Included (Fr and En)	
CISMeF	Included (Fr and En)	
Codes used for drugs	Included (Fr and En)	
DRC	Included (Fr and En)	
FMA	Included (Fr and En)	Included (En)
ICD10	Included (Fr and En)	Included (En)
IDIT	Included (Fr)	
IUPAC	Included (Fr and En)	
LOINC	Included (Partially translated Fr, En)	Included (En)
MedDRA	Included (Fr and En)	Included (Fr and En)
MEDLINEPlus	Included (Fr and En)	Included (En)
MeSH	Included (Fr and En)	Included (Fr and En)
NCCMERP	Included (En)	
ORPHANET	Included (Fr and En)	
PSIP Taxo.	Included (En)	
SNOMED International	Included (Fr and En)	Included (En)
UNIT	Included (Fr and En)	
VCM	Included (Fr)	
WHO-ART	Included (Fr and En)	Included (Fr and En)
WHO-ATC	Included (Fr and En)	
WHO-ICF	Included (Fr and En)	Included (En)
WHO-ICPC2	Included (Fr and En)	Included (Fr and En)
WHO-ICPS	Included (Fr and En)	

Table 1. List of the most represented terminologies included in the HMTP.

Terminologies	32
Terms/Concepts	980,000
Synonyms	2,300,00
Definitions	222,800
Relations and hierarchies	400,000

Table 2. Main figures of the Health Multi-Terminology Portal (November 2011).

Historically, the need for ontology alignment arose out of the need to integrate heterogeneous databases developed independently and thus each having their own data vocabulary. As terminology is a kind of ontology the definition of Euzenat stands for *Terminology Alignment*: the task of determining correspondences, i.e. alignments, between terms. Various studies have investigated automatic and semi-automatic methods and tools to map between medical terminologies to make them "interoperable" . The terminologies themselves are unaffected by the alignment process. Alignment techniques are of particular importance because the manual creation of correspondences between concepts or between terms is excessively time consuming. According to (Shvaiko & Euzenat, 2005) there are two major dimensions for similarity: the syntactic dimension and the semantic dimension. Syntactic dimension is based on lexical methods and semantic dimension is based on structural and semantic properties of terminologies (Euzenat & Shvaiko, 2007).

4.1.1 Lexical methods

Lexical methods are based on the lexical properties of terms. These methods are straightforward and represent a trivial approach to identifying correspondences between terms. The use of such methods in the medical domain to achieve mappings was motivated by the fact that most terminologies share many similar terms.

String-based Methods In these methods, terms or (labels) are considered as sequences of characters. A string distance is determined to compute a similarity degree. Some of these methods can skip the order of characters. Examples of such distances, also used in the context of information retrieval, are: the Hamming distance (Hamming, 1950), the Jaccard distance (Jaccard, 1901), Dice Distance (Salton & McGill, 1983). On the other hand, a family of appropriate measures known as "Edit distance", takes into account the order of characters. Intuitively, an edit distance between two strings is defined as being the minimum number of character inserts, deletes and changes needed to convert one string to another. Levenshtein distance (Levenshtein, 1966) is one example of such distances. It is the edit distance with all costs equal to 1. Another example of such distance is the SMOA distance (Stoilos et al., 2005) which is based on the idea that the similarity between two strings depends on their commonalities and differences. However, these methods can only quantify the similarity between terms or labels. Thus, they produce low (or no) similarity between synonyms term with different structures. For example, the two words "pain" and "Ache" are synonyms, *i.e.* related semantically as being the same thing, but all the distances presented above cannot identify any links between these two terms. Conversely, these methods find significant similarity between different terms (false positive), such as: "Vitamin A" and "Vitamin B".

Language-based Methods In these methods, terms are considered as words in a particular language. They rely on NLP tools to help the extraction of the meaningful terms from a text. These tools exploit morphological properties of words. We distinguish methods which are based on normalization process from those which exploit external knowledge resources such as dictionaries.

Normalization methods Each word is normalized to a standardized form that can be easily recognized. Several linguistic software tools are developed to quickly obtain a normal form of strings : (i) tokenization consists in segmenting strings into sequences of tokens by eliminating punctuation, cases, blank characters; (ii) the stemming process consists in analyzing the tokens derived in the tokenization process to reduce them to a canonical form; (iii) the stop words elimination consists in removing all the frequent short words that do not affect the sentences or the labels of terms, phrases such as "a", "Nos", "of"...etc

External-based methods These methods use external resources, such as dictionaries and lexicons. Several linguistic resources exists to found possible mappings between terminologies exist. These methods form the basis of the lexical tools used by the UMLSKS API (section 3.1). They were combined with synonyms from other external resources to optimize mapping to the UMLS. Another external resource largely used in the biomedical field is the lexical database WordNet (Fellbaum, 1998).

4.1.2 Semantic (or structural) methods

These methods use the structural properties of each terminology to identify possible correspondences between terms. They consider terminologies as graph were nodes represent terms and edge represent relations established in the terminology between these terms. Most medical terminologies can be represented as graph. Furthermore, these techniques can also be combined with lexšical techniques. The work presented in (Bodenreider et al., 1998) is a good example that illustrating the use of terminology relations to map terms not mapped with lexical methods. This algorithm used the semantic relationships between concepts from different terminologies included in the UMLS. In parallel with the structural properties of each terminology, semantic methods used also semantic similarities to find the closest term. The main technique consists in computing the number of edges between terms to determine a distance between them. The famous similarity distance is the Wu-Palmer distance (Wu & Palmer, 1994). This similarity is defined according to the distance between two terms in the hierarchy and also by their positions from the root. Unlike these traditional edge-counting approaches, other methods calculate the similarity according to the most information that two terms share in a hierarchical structure such as: Lin similarity (Lin, 1998) for example, this similarity was combined with a statistical similarity used to compute semantic similarity between CISMeF resources (Merabti et al., 2008). These similarities can be used to find possible connections between terms or concepts from different hierarchical terminologies, such MeSH or SNOMED Int for example.

4.2 Methods for evaluation of mapping results

Although fully automatic alignment might appear as the solution of choice for the interoperability of semantic systems, results provided by fully automatic methods are rarely of sufficient quality. In parallel to mapping methods, several techniques and methods were proposed to evaluate the mapping results produced by several systems. As defined in (Euzenat & Shvaiko, 2007), the goal of evaluation is to improve the mapping method and to give the user the best tool and method possible for the task. The main evaluation methods are based on the appropriateness and quality of the results, using a Likert scale or measures such as precision, recall, the F-measure and the of mapping. In (Ehrig & Euzenat, 2005) the authors proposed a framework for generalizing precision and recall and in (Euzenat, 2007) the author proposed a semantic precision and recall. These improvements were analyzed in (David & Euzenat, 2008) where more adaptations of these two measures to normalized mapping are proposed. In (Euzenat et al., 2011) one can find a panel of systems and results concerning the Ontology Alignment Evaluation Initiative. As in Information Retrieval systems evaluation, this type of evaluation needs a gold standard (GS) dataset. The problem is that these datasets are not available or easy to find or build as stated in (Euzenat et al., 2011). This is why the majority of evaluations used for our studies described hereafter are based on Likert scales where an expert manually evaluates a small set of mapping results according to specific levels. Nevertheless, the necessity of involving humans in the alignment process using visual interfaces has been outlined in (Kotis & Lanzenberger, 2008) within a discourse on ontology alignment challenges. On the same issue, as argued in (Granitzer et al., 2010) visual interfaces can address efficiently the problem of evaluating automatic alignment systems to take advantage of human cognitive capabilities and provide intuitive overview, navigation and detail analysis. Therefore, from next year we are going to offer to experts an evaluation tool connected to our databases to facilitate the evaluation of each automatic mapping. We think that regulated use of this tool can allow us to build a large dataset with valid and non valid mappings between terminologies that can be used to improve our methods.

5. Proposed methods for aligning medical terminologies

In this section we detail the methods we have developed for aligning terminologies included in the UMLS and HMTP described in section 3. We also detail the methods we have applied to evaluate the mapping results. Two automatic mapping approaches are implemented in the HMTP: conceptual and lexical approach. The former uses the UMLS Metathesaurus to map the terminologies included in the UMLS, whereas the latter exploits natural language processing tools to map terminologies whether or not they are included in the UMLS.

5.1 Conceptual approach

This approach is possible if each term to be mapped is included in the Metathesaurus (Joubert et al., 2009). The principle of the method is based on the conceptual construction of the UMLS Metathesaurus. Three types of mapping could be derived: "ExactMapping", "BroaderMapping" and/or "NarrowMapping" and "CloseMapping" (see Table 3 for examples). This method is inspired by the SKOS (Simple Knowledge Organization System) definitions of mapping properties[12]. Let t_1 and t_2 two terms belong to T_1 and T_2, two terminologies respectively. Suppose CUI_1 and CUI_2, the respective projections of t_1 and t_2 in the Metathesaurus, then t_1 and t_2 could be aligned if:

- $CUI_1 = CUI_2$, this corresponds to the "Exact Mapping".
- there is a parent of t_1 or t_2 which maps t_2 or t_1 respectively, this corresponds to "Broad Mapping" and/or "Narrow Mapping": these are used to state mapping links through hierarchies.
- there is explicit mapping between CUI_1 and CUI_2, this corresponds to the non-transitive "Close Mapping": two concepts are sufficiently similar that they can be used interchangeably.

The algorithm is carried out sequentially and stops when a candidate term for mapping is found. As an application of this, even if an explicit mapping comes from other terminologies in UMLS, e.g. ICD-9-CM and SNOMED CT (Imel, 2002) not part of terminologies under consideration, explicit mappings between two terminologies can be "reused" for other terminologies by using the UMLS concept structure (Fung & Bodenreider, 2005).

5.2 Lexical approach

In this approach, Natural Language Processing (NLP) tools adapted for the English and French languages) are used to link terms from different terminologies in the HMTP. The lexical approach allows us to find a term in the target terminology that is the most lexically similar to a given term in a source terminology.

---

[12] World Wide Web Consortium Simple Knowledge Organization System: www.w3.org/2004/02/skos

Type of relation	Source term (Terminology)	Target Term (Terminology)
Exact Mapping	Congenital bladder anomaly (MedDRA)	Congenital anomaly of the bladder, nos (SNMI)
Close Mapping	Diseases of lips (ICD10)	Ulcer of lip (SNMI)
BT-NT Mapping	Hepatic insufficiency (MeSH)	Liver disease, nos (ICPC2)

Table 3. Examples for each type of conceptual mapping.

5.2.1 Lexical approach for medical terminologies in French

This approach uses a French NLP tool and mapping algorithms developed by the CISMeF team to map French medical terminologies (Merabti, 2010; Merabti et al., 2010a;b). These tools were initially developed in previous works for information retrieval (Soualmia, 2004) and extended to link terms in multiple French medical terminologies:

- Remove stop words: frequent short words that do not affect the phrases such as "a", "Nos", "of", etc are removed from all terms in all terminologies in the HMTP.
- Stemming, a French stemmer provided by the "Lucene" software library which proved to be the most effective for automatic indexing using several health terminologies (Pereira, 2007). Mapping used by this approach may provide three types of alignments between all terms:
- Exact correspondence: if all words composing the two terms are exactly the same.
- Single to multiple correspondences: when the source term cannot be mapped by one exactly target term, but can be expressed by a combination of two or more terms.
- Partial correspondence: in this type of mapping only a part of the source term will be mapped to one or more target terms.

Examples for each type of mapping are given in Table 4. In this work, we describe only exact correspondences.

Type of correspondance	Source term (Terminology)	Target Term(s)(Terminology)
Exact	Syndrome de Marfan "Marfan Syndrome"(MeSH)	Syndrome de Marfan "Marfan's Syndrome" (MedDRA)
Single to Multiple	Albinisme surdité "Albinism- deafness syndrome" (ORPHANET)	Albinisme "Albinism" (MeSH) and (+) Surdité "Deafness" (SNMI)
Partial	Chromosome 14 en anneau "Ring chromosome 14" (ORPHANET)	Chromosome humain 14 "Chromosome 14" (MeSH)

Table 4. Examples of the three types of mappings using the French lexical approach.

5.2.2 Lexical approach for medical terminologies in English

In this approach we use lexical tools in English developed by the NLM (Browne et al., 2003) and included in the Lexical tool of the UMLS (see section 3.1). These tools were designed to aid users in analyzing and indexing natural language texts in the medical field (McCray et al., 1994; Peters et al., 2010). They include essentially :

- the LVG (Lexical Variant Generator): a Multi-function tool for lexical variation processing;
- Norm[13]: a program used to normalize English terminologies included in the UMLS ;
- WordInd: a tool used to tokenize terms into words.

In this work we have used the normalization program ("Norm"). The normalization process involves stripping genitive marks, transforming plural forms into singular, replacing punctuation, removing stop words, lower-casing each word, breaking a string into its constituent words, and sorting the words into alphabetic order. We have considered here only the exact correspondences. This type of mapping is easy to evaluate in English and the "not exact" correspondence will be useful for the translation of English terms into French. Several tools based on these techniques were used to map between medical terminologies. As an example, the authors in (Wang et al., 2008) used tokenisation and stemming techniques to map ICPS-2 with the SNOMED CT. It is also the case for the lexical techniques proposed by the NLM in the UMLSKS API. The NLM also created (Aronson, 2001) a tool to identify biomedical concepts from free textual input and map them into concepts from the UMLS. Authors in (Johnson et al., 2006) used the Lucene API to found relations between Gene Ontology (GO) and three other biomedical ontologies.

5.3 Structural approach

This approach is based on hierarchical relations and was used to align the remaining terms not mapped by the lexical approach. This mapping provides two types of correspondences:

- BroadMapping: when the remaining term has at least one parent (hierarchical relation broader than) mapped to at least one term.
- NarrowMapping: when the remaining term has at least one child (hierarchical relation narrower than) mapped to at least one term.

The work presented in (Bodenreider & McCray, 1998) is a good example that illustrates the use of the terminology relations to map terms not mapped with the lexical methods. This algorithm exploit the semantic relationships between concepts from different terminologies included in the UMLS.

6. Cases studies

In this section we present some cases of alignments between medical terminologies, essentially in French, to the UMLS, HMTP or other terminologies.

---

[13] National Library of Medicine: Lexical Tools:
http://lexsrv3.nlm.nih.gov/LexSysGroup/Projects/lvg/2010/docs/userDoc/index.html

6.1 Aligning the ORPHANET thesaurus to the MeSH thesaurus

In order to align the ORPHANET thesaurus, which describes rare diseases to the MeSH thesaurus, we have compared two methods. The first one uses the UMLS and an external manual alignment of ORPHANET terms to ICD10 codes. The second one uses only lexical-based approach without using the UMLS to make a direct and an automatic alignment between ORPHANET and MeSH. We also provide an evaluation and a comparison of these two methods. The MeSH thesaurus was chosen as the target terminology for comparing alignment strategies for two main reasons:

- the ORPHANET team needs to map each ORPHANET term to a MeSH term to allow a contextual link between an ORPHANET Web page for one ORPHANET rare disease (e.g. Marfan syndrome) and one corresponding PubMed query. The CISMeF team has strong experience with the MeSH thesaurus. Therefore, the evaluation will conducted done by a CISMeF expert.

- the MeSH thesaurus is the second largest terminology available represented in the UMLS and it freely available in the HMTP. Nevertheless, ORPHANET is now aligned to all French and English terminologies available in the HMTP and several relations from this terminology are also available (not freely) in the HMTP.

6.1.1 Methods

The first method "Manual ORPHANET-ICD10 link-based alignment" is based on the external manual alignment between ORPHANET and ICD10 terms performed by the ORPHANET team. In this approach, the link provided by the UMLS Metathesaurus between ICD10 and MeSH is used. Hence, an effective alignment exists between two terms ICD10 and MeSH if these terms share the same UMLS Concept Unique Identifier (CUI) in the Metathesaurus. For example, there is an effective alignment between the ICD10 term "Cushing syndrome" (Code: E24) and the MeSH term "Cushing syndrome" since they share the same UMLS Concept CUI: C0010481)(Table 5).

ORPHANET Term	ICD10 term	MeSH term
Cushing syndrome	SCushing's syndrome	Cushing Syndrome
Ichthyosis, X-linked	X-linked ichthyosis	Ichthyoses, X-Linked
Muscular dystrophy, Duchenne and Becker types	Muscular dystrophy	Muscular Dystophies

Table 5. Example of UMLS and manual ORPHANET-ICD10 links based mapping.

The second method is the "Lexical-based alignment" which is described in the section 5.2 This method allows us to find a term in the target terminology (MeSH) that is the most lexically similar, from a given term in the source terminology (ORPHANET). We have however also used a structural approach to align the remaining ORPHANET terms to the MeSH.

6.1.2 Evaluation & comparison

To evaluate the two methods, four sets of correspondences were derived from the results of the two methods applied to 2,083 ORPHANET terms manually aligned to the ICD10:

- First set: The correspondences obtained by the first strategy "UMLS and manual ORPHANET ICD10 link-based alignment" and not by the second "lexical-based approach" (only manually found)
- Second set: The correspondences found by the second method and not by the first (Only Lexical-based mapping found)
- Third set: The discrepant correspondences found by both methods for the same ORPHANET term. For example, for the ORPHANET term "Tangier disease" the two methods found two different MeSH terms, the MeSH term "Hypolipoprotenemia" with the first method and the MeSH term "Tangier disease" with the second.
- Fourth set: The correspondences found with both methods (the same correspondences).

A sample of 100 correspondences, randomly determined, from each set was evaluated by a physician (SJD), head of the CISMeF team. The following terms were used to describe the quality of each mapping result: (i)"relevant" the mapping between one MeSH term and one ORPHANET term was rated as correct; (ii) "non-relevant" when the mapping between MeSH and ORPHANET terms was considered by the expert as not correct; (iii) "BT-NT" the ORPHANET term was rated as broader than the MeSH corresponding term; (iv) "NT-BT" the ORPHANET term was rated as narrower than the MeSH corresponding term. For example, "Duchenne and Becker muscular dystrophy" is narrower than "muscular dystrophies" and (v) "Sibling" when the MeSH corresponding and ORPHANET term are siblings (from the MeSH point of view). For example, "Cryptophthalmia, isolated" is evaluated as the sibling of "microphthalmos".

6.1.3 Results

For the UMLS and manual ORPHANET-ICD10 link-based alignment: Among the 2,083 ORPHANET terms (28% of all ORPHANET terms) manually aligned to at least one ICD10 code, 619 possible correspondences were found for at least one MeSH term using the UMLS (30% from 2,083). For the lexical-based approach (only limited to the ORPHANET terms manually linked to ICD10), among the 2,083 ORPHANET terms linked manually to at least one ICD10 code, 593 possible correspondences were found for at least one MeSH term (28% from 2,083). However, 1,004 possible correspondences were found to at least one MeSH term (13% from 7,424) when this method was applied to the whole ORPHANET thesaurus. According to the results of each method we obtained:

1. The first set contains 327 correspondences were found only by the "UMLS and manual ORPHANET ICD10 manual alignments" and not by the "lexical-based alignment".
2. The second set contains the 306 correspondences were found only by the "lexical-based alignment".
3. The third set contains the 75 different correspondences were found by both methods with the same ORPHANET term.
4. The fourth set contains the 211 same correspondences were found by both methods.

The results of the evaluation of the correspondences obtained by each strategy independently are displayed in Table 6. Overall 85% of correspondences obtained by method 2 (Lexical-based mapping) are ranked as relevant when only 21% of correspondences are ranked as relevant for the first strategy (UMLS and manual ORPHANET-ICD10 link-based alignment), whereas 32% and 15% of the correspondences obtained by methods 1 and 2 respectively are ranked as NT-BT (the source term is evaluated as narrower than the target term in the MeSH hierarchy). Table 7 displays the evaluation results for the third set containing different correspondences from the two strategies for the same ORPHANET term. For the first strategy (UMLS and manual Orphanet-ICD10 link-based alignment), overall 39 correspondences are evaluated as "BT-NT" when only 6 correspondences are evaluated as "relevant". For the second method (Lexical-based mapping), overall there are 62 correspondences evaluated as "relevant", whereas 8 correspondences are evaluated as "BT-NT". The results of evaluation for the fourth set containing the same correspondences derived by each method found relevant correspondences in 98% cases and BT-NT relations in 2% cases.

	Relevant	BT-NT	NT-BT	Sibling	Non-relevant
First Set	21	2	32	0	45
Second Set	85	0	15	0	0

Table 6. Evaluation results of the two sets of correspondences (correspondences found by each strategy only).

	Relevant	BT-NT	NT-BT	Sibling	Non-relevant
UMLS and manual ORPHANET-ICD10 link-based mapping	6	39	7	2	21
Lexical-based alignement	62	8	1	1	2

Table 7. Evaluation results of the fourth set of correspondences (for the same ORPHANET term different correspondences).

Using a lexical-based approach (to all HMTP) 4,669 ORPHANET terms were aligned to at least one terminology from the HMTP. From this set of correspondences, 1,433 ORPHANET terms were aligned with at least one MeSH term (30%). On the other hand, from the remaining ORPHANET terms the structural alignments between ORPHANET and all the terms from HMTP provided: 1,513 ORPHANET terms in broader correspondence and 957 ORPHANET terms in NT correspondence. An ORPHANET expert has evaluated the two correspondences: lexical-based and structural. From 100 lexical-based alignments, 99% were evaluated as relevant and from 500 structural alignments 482 were evaluated as relevant, when 16 were evaluated as irrelevant.

6.2 Aligning the CCAM to the UMLS

The objective of this section is to describe an alignment method that may be used to integrate any medical terminology in French in the UMLS Metathesaurus. The alignment method has been used and evaluated to align the CCAM terminology (Classification Commune des Actes Médicaux) for procedures to the UMLS Metathesaurus. The CCAM is a multi-hierarchical structured classification for mainly surgical procedures used in France for reimbursement and policymaking in health care. Each procedure is described by a code using "CCAM Basic

Coding System", which consists of coding: (1) body system/anatomical site or function, (2) action and (3) approach/method (see the Table 8).

NC	Bones of the leg
C	Osteosynthesis
A	Open Approach
NCCA010	Osteosynthesis of tibial diaphysis fracture by external fixing

Table 8. Example of CCAM basic coding.

6.2.1 Method

The alignment method for mapping CCAM codes to UMLS concepts is based on the structure of the CCAM codes. However, it is impossible to assign one or more specific UMLS concept using only CCAM labels. This is mainly due to the length of CCAM labels. Indeed, there are 85% of CCAM labels that are composed of 5 or more than 5 words vs. only 5% of the MeSH descriptors. In this approach, only the first significant three characters that compose the CCAM code according to the anatomic and action axes are aligned with the UMLS Metathesaurus. For example, the CCAM code "MZQH001" that has the label "Arthrography of upper limb with scanography [Arthroscan ofupper limb]", is represented according to the first significant three characters with "Bones, joints and soft tissues of upper limb, multiple locations or not specified + Arthrography". In this context we have used the lexical-based method described in section 5.2 to align the first three characters of each CCAM code. This alignment provides three types of correspondences between all terms in source terminologies and French terms of the UMLS Metathesaurus: (i) exact, (ii) Single to multiple and (iii) partial(see Table 9).

CCAM code	Anatomic axis	Action axis	Corresponding term	Type of mapping
BDHA001	Cornea	biopsy	Biopsy cornea	Exact
AAFA003	Brain	exeresis	Brain and Exeresis	Single to multiple
DGFA013	Aorta	laparotomie	Aorte	Partial correspondance

Table 9. Examples of the three types of mappings using the lexical-based approach.

6.2.2 Evaluation

Evaluation was performed on all correspondences from the "exact" set and for only 100 correspondences from the "Single to multiple" set. We chose only 100 mappings because in most cases the same codes with the same first three characters are mapped to the same terms (HLHH003, HLHH004…). Qualitative evaluation was performed by a physician, expert in CCAM codes and in UMLS. The following terms were used to rate the quality of each correspondence: (i) "equivalent" the UMLS concept corresponds exactly to the CCAM code; (ii) "BT-NT" when the CCAM code was rated as broader than the UMLS concept according to the label of the CCAM and the preferred terms (PTs) in the UMLS concepts; (iii) "NT-BT" the CCAM code was rated as narrower than the PTs in the UMLS concept; (iv) "incomplete" when the UMLS concept only reflects some part of the CCAM label and (v) "irrelevant" when the correspondence was considered by the expert as incorrect. For example, the correspondence between the CCAM code "HLFA001" (label: "Right hepatectomy, by laparotomy") and the UMLS concept C0193399 (preferred term: "Lobectomy of liver") was rated as NT-BT because the UMLS concept is narrow and less precise than the CCAM label. However, for the "Single to multiple" set, the expert performed the evaluation in two steps: (1) each pair (CCAM axe, UMLS concept) is evaluated independently and (2) the correspondence between the CCAM code and the combination of the UMLS concepts is evaluated in this second phase. For example, evaluating the correspondence between the CCAM code "AAFA003" and the two UMLS concepts: C006104 (preferred term: "Brain") and C0919588 ((preferred term: "Exeresis"), (i) first, the expert evaluates each axe with corresponding UMLS ((Brain, C006104) =equivalent and (Exeresis, C091958) =equivalent)); (ii) second, the expert evaluates the correspondence between the label and the combination of the two UMLS concepts (AAFA003, (C006104, C091958) =NT-BT).

6.2.3 Results

Using this method, there are 5,212 (65%) CCAM codes out of the 7,926 CCAM codes used in this study that provide possible correspondences from the CCAM to French terms in the UMLS. The results of each type of correspondence are displayed in Table 10. There are 2,210 (27.5%) correspondences according to both the anatomic and action axes. In the other hand, there are 1,716 (21%) correspondences according to the anatomic axis alone and 1,286 (16%) correspondences according to the action axis. Overall, 65% of the correspondences "anatomic terms" in the CCAM codes are aligned to at least one UMLS Concept and 37% of the correspondences "action terms" in the CCAM codes are aligned to at least one UMLS Concept. For the set of exact correspondences (n=200), 182 (91%) correspondences between CCAM codes and UMLS concepts were rated as NT-BT and only in 9 cases where they rated as equivalent (see Table 11). For the set of single to multiple correspondences (n=100), 61 (61%) and 44 (44%) of the anatomic and the action axes respectively are equivalent to at least one UMLS concept. According to this type of correspondence, 27 (27%) correspondences between CCAM code and at least one UMLS concept were rated as exactly equivalent, when 54 were rated as NT-BT (see Table 12).

Type of mapping	Number of mappings
Exact	200(2.5%)
Single to multiple	2,010(25%)
"Exact" Partial mapping	3,002(37.8%)

Table 10. Results of each correspondence type.

Relevant	BT-NT	NT-BT	Incomplete	Irrelevant	Total
9 (4.5%)	0 (0%)	182 (91%)	3 (1.5%)	6 (3%)	200

Table 11. Evaluation results of the "exact" correspondence set.

Single to multiple mapping	Equivalent	BT-NT	NT-BT	Incomplete	irrelevant
Anatomic	61 (61%)	1 (1%)	29 (29%)	9 (9%)	0 (0%)
Action	44 (44%)	0 (0%)	49 (49%)	1(1%)	6 (6%)
Combination	27 (27%)	0 (0%)	54 (54%)	10 (10%)	9 (9%)

Table 12. Evaluation results of the "Single to Multiple" correspondence set (n=100).

7. Global results

7.1 Conceptual approach

There are 199,786 correspondences exist between at least two French terms from UMLS (25,833 (ExactMapping), 69,085 (CloseMapping) and 104,868 (Broader and /or NarrowerMapping)). In contrast, from the 25,833 terms rated "Exactly", 15,831 come from SNOMED International whereas only 296 come from ICPC2 (Table 13). The three types of correspondences ("Exact", "Broader" and/or "Narrow" and "Close") are included in the HMTP (see Figure 1).

Terminology	Number of terms mapped
ICD10	3,282 (35%)
ICPC2	296 (39%)
MedDRA	5,700 (28%)
MeSH	10,637 (40%)
SNOMED Int.	15,831 (14%)
WHO-ART	1,392 (81%)

Table 13. Number of terms from each terminology having exact correspondence (conceptual approach).

7.2 Lexical approach

There are 266,139 correspondences exist between at least two terms of the HMTP (English and French). However, the majority of correspondences have not yet been evaluated. Terminologies included in the HMTP in English and French were aligned using the two lexical approaches. Table 14 displays a fragment of the entire matrix mapping between all terminologies of the HMTP. For example, the MeSH, SNOMED International, ORPHANET and ATC terminologies were aligned using English and French lexical approaches. However, some terminologies were mapped using an English (SNOMED CT, PSIP Taxonomy) or French (CISMeF, DRC) lexical approach alone. All exact correspondences were integrated into the HMTP (Figure 2).

8. Use of alignments

8.1 Alignments for information retrieval

8.1.1 Information retrieval

Thanks to the multiple inter and intra terminology relations derived, the information retrieval results can be improved and can better respond to user's queries through "query expansion"

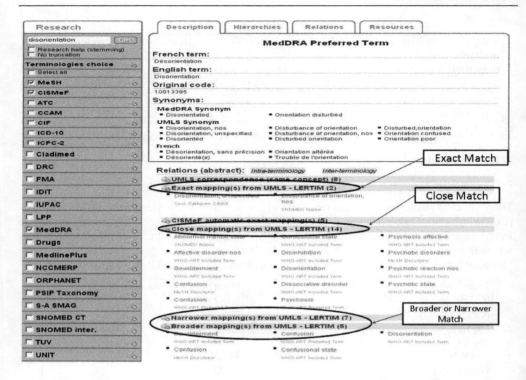

Fig. 1. The three types of conceptual approach integrated into the HMTP (Example of the MedDRA term "Disorientation").

or "query reformulation". Inter and Intra relations will be used to ensure navigation between terminologies. Thus, we can find all the possible connections between the terms of query in a given terminology and all other terms in other terminologies. This process can widen the scope of the search for the user according to its context without impacting the relevance of the information or the precision of the system. For example, according to the mapping between the MeSH term "Hearing aids" and the SNOMED Int term "Auditory system" we can expand the results and return all resources indexed by both terms.

8.1.2 InfoRoute

InfoRoute (Darmoni et al., 2008) is a French Infobutton (Cimino et al., 1997) developed by CISMeF. It allows the search of the main institutional websites to access high-quality documents available in French on the Internet. The CISMeF team selected fifty websites produced by high-quality Internet publishers (Figure 3), such as governments from French-speaking countries (France, Switzerland, Belgium, Canada and many African countries), national health agencies, medical societies and medical schools. Health documents on the Internet may be accessed through their description with the MeSH thesaurus: MEDLINE bibliographic database, French CISMeF, Australian Healthinsite, UK Intute catalogs. Therefore, the use of correspondences between MeSH and all terminologies used

	FMA	MedDRA	MeSH	ORPHANET	SNOMED Int	WHO-ART
CCAM	0	110	305	0	430	5
CISMeF	9	99	517	11	222	17
CISP2	7	138	219	30	254	109
Codes for drugs	0	24	1,455	3	302	0
FMA		119	1,745	32	5,777	3
ICD10	10,209	2,380	3,827	947	7,474	1,134
MedDRA	119		3,728	885	5,360	1,278
MEDLINEPlus	34	314	675	138	448	170
MeSH	1,745	3,728		1,805	15,127	1,417
ORPHANET	32	885	1,805		1,635	284
SNOMED Int	5,777	5,360	15,127	1,635		1,747
WHO-ART	3	1,278	1,417	284	1,747	
WHO-ATC	61	58	3,533	0	1,581	4
WHO-ICF	178	9	294	2	222	7
WHO-ICPS	1	13	159	0	114	6

Table 14. Fragment of the entire matrix mapping from HMTP.

to index documents in these websites is a good solution. For example: MeSH to ORPHANET (ORPHANET website), MeSH to MEDLINEplus Topics (MEDLINEPlus).

8.2 Alignments for translation

Methods developed to align biomedical terminologies were also used to translate automatically several biomedical terminologies. For example in (Deléger et al., 2010) we have combined the UMLS-based approach (conceptual approach) and a corpus-based approach to translate MEDLINEPlus® Topics from English into French. The first method based on the conceptual approach brought translations for 611 terms (from 848 MEDLINEPlus PT), 67% of which were considered valid. In (Merabti et al., 2011), we have compared two methods to translate the FMA terms into French. The first one used the conceptual approach based on conceptual information from the UMLS Metathesaurus. The two approaches allowed semi-automatic translation of 3,776 FMA terms from English into French, which was added to the existing 10,844 French FMA terms in the HMTP (4,436 FMA French terms and 6,408 FMA terms manually translated). The same approaches were used to translate 114,917 SNOMED CT English terms (40%) to at least one French term. For the FMA translation for example, evaluation methods demonstrated that 59% of the translations were rated as "good" for lexical approach and 69% for the conceptual approach. These approaches are integrated into the HMTP to translate automatically English terms to French. However, to improve the quality of the trans-lation a manual validation is needed in parallel of this automatic processing.

9. Discussion

In this chapter, we have presented the problem of integrating heterogeneous sources of medical terminologies such as thesauri, classifications, nomenclatures or controlled vocabularies to allow semantic interoperability between systems. Terminology alignment is the task of creating links between two original terminologies. These links could be

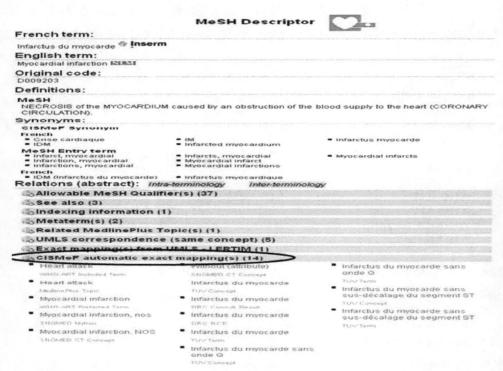

Fig. 2. Mapping of the MeSH term "myocardial infarction" according to the lexical approach in HMTP (Exact correspondence).

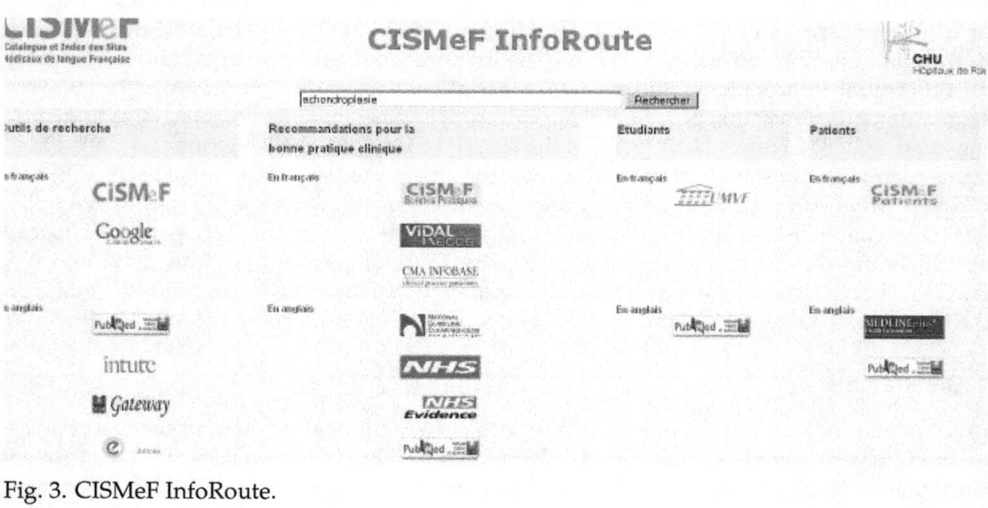

Fig. 3. CISMeF InfoRoute.

equivalences, correspondences or relations between terms and concepts having the same meaning but expressed with different labels. We have also presented the main methods that are commonly used for alignment between ontologies and show how we have derived them for medical terminologies. Structural methods are independent of language but the lexical ones we have presented stand for medical terminologies expressed in English and French. We have also proposed a method for evaluating sets of correspondences. All the sets of correspondences and relations we have derived are used in different contexts of information retrieval through the CISMeF catalogue and accessed through the Health Multiple Teminologies Portal developed at Rouen University Hospital. The essential difference between the alignments included in the HMTP and BioPortal (Ghazvinian et al., 2009a) is that the latter has applied lexical matching of preferred names and synonyms in English to generate alignments between concepts in BioPortal ontologies. Thus, they may miss a connection between two ontologies that actually have a significant amount of overlap in terms of the actual concepts they represent simply because these concepts have different lexical structures in the two ontologies. However, users can browse the correspondences, create new correspondences, upload correspondences created with other tools, download the correspondences stored in BioPortal, or comment on them and discuss them. Many works on aligning medical terminologies have been published recently showing that it is an active research area. In (Alecu et al., 2006), when mapping MedDRA to SNOMED CT instead of considering an unmapped MedDRA term, they considered its mapped ancestor by exploiting hierarchical relations (structure level approach). In (Bodenreider, 2009) when mapping SNOMED CT to MedDRA hierarchical relations from SNOMED CT, which are far more fine-grained than those from MedDRA, were exploited and enabled on the whole over 100 000 new mappings. However these two studies attempted to find correspondences of MedDRA terms as such, without completing the approach from a lexical standpoint trying for example to decompose and then align them to more than one SNOMED CT term. Indeed, in (Ghazvinian et al., 2009b) the comparison of different alignment approaches for medical terminologies shows that simple lexical methods perform best since medical terminologies have strongly controlled vocabularies and share little structure. Finally a specific browser was designed in order to align frequent MedDRA terms with SNOMED CT terms (Nadkarni & Darer, 2010). It was enriched with simple synonyms from the UMLS and considered decompositions of MedDRA terms. In (Diosan et al., 2009) the authors propose an automatic method for aligning different definitions taken from general dictionaries that could be associated with the same medical term although they may have the same label. The terms are those included in the CISMeF database. The method used is based on classification by Support Vector Machines derived from methods for aligning sentences from bilingual corpora (Moore, 2002). In (Milicic Brandt et al., 2011) the authors present a similar method for creating mappings between the ORPHANET thesaurus of rare diseases and the UMLS, mainly for aligning it with SNOMED CT, the MeSH thesaurus and MedDRA. The authors also use the lexical tool Norm included in the UMLS Lexical Tools to normalize terminologies included in the UMLS and normalize the ORPHANET thesaurus by "aggressive" normalization adding more steps in the process for example removing further stop words such as "disease" or "disorder". In (Mougin et al., 2011) the authors present a method for mapping MedDRA and SNOMED CT via the UMLS. They propose an automatic lexical-based approach with normalization, segmentation and tokenization steps. This approach is completed by filtering terms according to the UMLS Semantic Network: if mapping is exact but the terms do not belong to the same Semantic Type, the resulting mapping is eliminated from the sets of mappings to be evaluated. However, this method of filtering cannot be applied when a terminology is not included in the UMLS. The evaluation in this study is quantitative and qualitative and the aim was to explore adverse drug reactions in clinical reports. Nonetheless, these correspondences are not used in concrete applications that propose semantic interoperability between systems such as the HMTP.

10. Conclusion

To summarize, we were able to achieve automatic alignment between Biomedical Terminologies. The methods we have proposed be applied to map English or French terms. The results obtained through these methods differ according to type of terminology and number of target terms used to map the source terminology. These methods are also used to translate some English terminologies to French (SNOMED CT, MEDLINEPlus).

11. Acknowledgements and funding

Multi-terminology portal was supported in part by the grants InterSTIS project (ANR-07-TECSAN-010);   ALADIN   project   (ANR-08-TECS-001);   L3IM   project (ANR-08-TECS-00); PSIP project; (Patient Safety through Intelligent Procedures in medication -FP7-ICT-2007-); PlaIR project, funded by FEDER. The authors thank Nikki Sabourin (Rouen University Hospital) for her valuable advice in editing the manuscript.

12. References

Alecu, I., Bousquet, C., Mougin, F. & Jaulent, M. (2006). Mapping of the whoÛart terminology on snomed ct to improve grouping of related adverse drug reactions, *Stud Health Inform* 124: 833–838.

Aronson, A. (2001). Effective mapping of biomedical text to the UMLS metathesaurus: the MetaMap program, *AMIA Annu Symp Proc*, pp. 17–21.

Aymé, S., Urbero, B., Oziel, D., Lacouturier, E. & Biscarat, A. (1998). Information on rare diseases: the ORPHANET project, *Rev Med Interne* 19(Suppl 3): 376S–377S.

Bodenreider, O. (2004). The Unified Medical Language System (UMLS): Integrating biomedical terminology, *Nucleic Acids Res* 32: 267–270.

Bodenreider, O. (2009). Using snomed ct in combination with meddra for reporting signal detection and adverse drug reactions reporting, *AMIA Ann Symp Proceedings*.

Bodenreider, O. & McCray, A. T. (1998). From french vocabulary to the unified medical language system: a preliminary study., *Stud Health Technol Inform* 52 Pt 1: 670–674.

Bodenreider, O., Nelson, S. J., Hole, W. T. & Chang, H. F. (1998). Beyond synonymy: exploiting the UMLS semantics in mapping vocabularies, *Proc. AMIA Symp. 1998*, pp. 815–819.

Brown, E., Wood, L. & Wood, S. (1999). The Medical Dictionary for Regulatory Activities (MedDRA), *Drug Safety* 2: 109–117.

Browne, A., G, D., Aronson, A. & AT, M. (2003). Umls language and vocabulary tools, *AMIA Annu Symp Proc*, p. 798.

Chute, C., Elkin, P., Sheretz, D. & Tuttle, M. (1999). Desiderata for a clinical terminology server, *Proc. AMIA Symp. 1999*, pp. 42–6.

Cimino, J., Elhanan, G. & Zeng, Q. (1997). Supporting Infobuttons with terminoligical knowledge, *JAMIA* 4(Suppl): 528–532.

Cormont, S., Vandenbussche, P., Buemi, A., Delahousse, J., Lepage, E. & Charlet, J. (2011). Implementation of a platform dedicated to biomedical analysis terminologies management, *Proc. AMIA Annu Symp Proc.*

Cornet, R. & de Keizer, N. (2008). Forty years of SNOMED: a literature review, *BMC Medical Informatics and Decision Making* 8(Suppl 1): S2.

Côté, R. A., Rothwell, D. J., Patolay, J., Beckett, R. & Brochu, L. (1993). The Systematised Nomenclature of Human and Veterinary Medicine: SNOMED International.

Darmoni, S. J., Joubert, M., Dahamna, B., Delahousse, J. & Fieschi, M. (2009a). SMTS: a French Health Multi-Terminology Server, p. 808.

Darmoni, S. J., Pereira, S., Névéol, A., Massari, P., Dahamna, B., Letord, C., Kerdelhué, G., Piot, J., Derville, A. & Thirion, B. (2008). French infobutton: an academic and business perspective., *AMIA Annu Symp Proc* p. 920.

Darmoni, S., Sakji, S., Pereira, S., Merabti, T., Prieur, E., Joubert, M. & Thirion, B. (2009b). Multiple terminologies in an health portal: automatic indexing and information retrieval, *Artificial Intelligence in Medicine*, Lecture Notes in Computer Science, Springer, Verona, Italy, pp. 255–259.

David, J. & Euzenat, J. (2008). On fixing semantic alignment evaluation measures, *The Third International Workshop on Ontology Matching*.

Deléger, L., Merabti, T., Lecroq, T., Joubert, M., Zweigenbaum, P. & Darmoni, S. (2010). A Twofold Strategy for Translation a Medical Terminology into French, *Proc. AMIA Symp. 2010*, pp. 152–6.

Diosan, L., Rogozan, A. & Pécuchet, J. (2009). *Automatic Alignment of Medical Terminologies with General Dictionaries for an Efficient Information Retrieval*, IGI Publisher, chapter 5, pp. 78–105.

Doan, A., Noy, N. & Halvey, A. (2004). Introduction to the special issue on semantic integration, *SIGMOD Record* 33: 11–13.

Douyère, M., Soualmia, L. F., Névéol, A., Rogozan, A., Dahamna, B., Leroy, J.-P., Thirion, B. & Darmoni, S. J. (2004). Enhancing the MeSH thesaurus to retrieve French online health resources in a quality-controlled gateway., *Health Info Libr J* 21(4): 253–261.

Ehrig, M. & Euzenat, J. (2005). Relaxed precision and recall for ontology matching, *Integrating Ontologies Workshop*.

Euzenat, J. (2007). Semantic precision and recall for ontology alignement evaluation, *IJCAI*.

Euzenat, J., Meilicke, C., Stuckenschmidt, H., Shvaiko, P. & Trojahn, C. (2011). Ontology alignment evaluation initiative: six years of experience, *Journal on Data Semantics* .

Euzenat, J. & Shvaiko, P. (2007). *Ontology Matching*, Hiedelberg: Springer-Varlag.

Fellbaum, C. (ed.) (1998). *WordNet: an electronic lexical database*, MIT Press.

Ferru, P. & Kandel, O. (2003). Dictionnaire des résultats de consultation (révision 2003-04), *Doc Rech Med Gen* 62: 3–54.

Fung, K. & Bodenreider, O. (2005). Utilizing UMLS for semantic mapping between terminologies, *Proc AMIA Symp*, pp. 266–270.

Ghazvinian, A., Noy, N., Jonquet, C., Shah, N. & Musen, M. (2009a). What four million mappings can tell you about two hundred ontologies, *Proceedings of the 8th ISWC*.

Ghazvinian, A., Noy, N. & Musen, M. (2009b). Creating mappings for ontologies in biomedicine: Simple methods work, *AMIA Annual Symposium*.

Granitzer, M., Sabol, V., Onn, K., Lukose, D. & Tochtermann, K. (2010). Ontology alignement-A Survey with focus on visually supported semi-automatic techniques, *Future Internet* 2(3): 238–258.

Grosjean, J., Merabti, T., Dahamna, B., Kergouraly, I. & Thirion, B. (2011). Health Multi-Terminology Portal: a semantic added-value for partient safety, *Patient Safety Informatics - Adverse Drug Events, Human Factors and IT*, Vol. 166, pp. 129–138.

Gruber, T. (1993). Toward principles for the design of ontologies used for knowledge sharing, *Formal Ontology in Conceptual Analysis and Knowledge Representation*, Kluwar Academic Publishers.

Hamming, R. (1950). Error detecting and error correcting codes, *Technical report*, Bell System Technical Journal.

Imel, M. (2002). A closer look: the SNOMED clinical terms to ICD-9-CM mapping., *J AHIMA* 73(6): 66–9; quiz 71–2.

Jaccard, J. (1901). Distribution de la flore alpine dans le bassin des dranses et dans quelques régions voisines, *Bulletin de la société vaudoise des sciences naturelles* 37: 241–272.

Johnson, H., Cohen, K., Baumgartner, W., Lu, Z., Bada, M., Kester, T., Kim, H. & Hunter, L. (2006). Evaluation of lexical methods for detecting relationships between concepts from multiple ontologies, *Pacific Symposium on Biocomputing*.

Joubert, M., Abdoune, H., Merabti, T., Darmoni, S. & Fieschi, M. (2009). Assisting the translation of SNOMED CT into French using UMLS and four representative French-language terminologies, *Proc. AMIA Symp.*, pp. 291–295.

Kotis, K. & Lanzenberger, M. (2008). Ontology matching: current status, dilemmas and future challenges, *International Conference on Complex, Intelligent and Software Intensive Systems*, pp. 924–927.

Lamy, J.-B., Ducols, C., Bar-Hen, A., Ouvrard, P. & Venot, A. (2008). An iconic language for the graphical representation of medical concepts, *BMC Bioinformatics* 8: 16.

Lefevre, P. (2000). *La recherche d'informations : du texte intégral au thésaurus*, Editions Hermès.

Levenshtein, V. I. (1966). Binary codes capable of correcting deletions, insertions and reversals, *Sov. Phys. Dokl.* pp. 707–710.

Lin, D. (1998). An information-theoretic definition of similarity, *Proc. Int. Conf. on Machine Learning*, pp. 296–304.

Lindberg, D. A., Humphreys, B. L. & McCray, A. T. (1993). The unified medical language system., *Methods Inf Med* 32(4): 281–291.

McCray, A., Srinivasan, S. & Brown, A. (1994). Lexical methods for managing variation in biomedical terminologies, *Annual Symposium on Computer Applications in Medical Care*, pp. 235–239.

Merabti, T. (2010). *Methods to map health terminologies: contribution to the semantic interoperability between health terminologies*, PhD thesis, University of Rouen.

Merabti, T., Joubert, M., Lecroq, T., Rath, A. & Darmoni, S. (2010a). Mapping biomedical terminologies using natural language processing tools and UMLS: mapping the Orphanet thesaurus to the MeSH, *Biomedical Engineering and Research* 31(4): 221–225.

Merabti, T., Massari, P., Joubert, M., Sadou, E., Lecroq, T., Abdoune, H., Rodrigues, J. & Darmoni, S. (2010b). Automated approach to map a French terminology to UMLS, *MedInfo2010*, Vol. 160, Cap Town, South Africa, pp. 1040–1044.

Merabti, T., Pereira, S., Letord, C., Lecroq, T., Dahamna, B., Joubert, M. & Darmoni, S. (2008). Searching related resources in a quality controlled health gateway: a feasibility study, *The XXIst International Congress of the European Federation for Medical Informatics (MIE'08)*, Vol. 136, pp. 235–249.

Merabti, T., Soualmia, L. F., Grosjean, J., Palombi, O., Müller, J.-M. & Darmoni, S. J. (2011). Translating the Foundational Model of Anatomy into French using knowledge-based and lexical methods, *BMC Medical Informatics and Decision Making* 11: 65.

Milicic Brandt, M., Rath, A., A., D. & S., A. (2011). Mapping orphanet terminology to umls, *Proceedings of 13th Conference on Artificial Intelligence in MEdicine, AIME*, p. 194Û203.

Miller, N., Lacroix, E. M. & Backus, J. E. (2000). MEDLINEplus: building and maintaining the national library of medecine's consumer health web service, *Bull Med Libr Assoc* 88(1): 11–7.

Moore, R. (2002). Machine translation: From research to real users, *Proceedings of ATMA, Lecture Notes in Computer Science*, Vol. 2499, pp. 135–144.

Mougin, F., Dupuch, M. & Grabar, N. (2011). Improving the mapping between meddra and snomed ct, *Proceedings of 13th Conference on Artificial Intelligence in MEdicine*.

Nadkarni, P. & Darer, J. (2010). Determining correspondences between high frequency meddra concepts and snomed: a case study, *BMC Med Infor. Decis. Mak* 10: 66.

Nelson, S., Johnston, D. & Humphreys, B. (2001). *Relationships in Medical Subject Headings*, New York: Kluwer Academic Publishers, pp. 171–184.

Noy, N., Musen, M., Mejino, J. L. & Rosse, C. (2004). Pushing the envelope: challenges in a frame-based representation, *Data Knowl. Eng.* 48: 335–359.

Pereira, S. (2007). *Muti-Terminology indexing of concepts in health*, PhD thesis, University of Rouen.

Pereira, S., Névéol, A., Kerdelhué, G., Serrot, E., Joubert, M. & Darmoni, S. J. (2008). Using multi-terminology indexing for the assignment of MeSH descriptors to health resources in a French online catalogue., *AMIA Annu Symp Proc* pp. 586–590.

Peters, L., Kapusnik-Uner, J. & Bodenreider, O. (2010). Methods for managing variation in clinical drug names, *Proc Annu Symp AMIA 2010*, pp. 637–4.

Rector, A., Bechhover, S. & Goble, C. (1997). The GRAIL concept modelling language for medical terminology, *Artif Intell Med* 9(2): 139–71.

Robinson, P. & Mundlos, S. (2010). The human phenotype ontology, *Clin Genet* 77: 525–534.

Roche, C. (2005). Terminologie et ontologie, *Revue Langages* 157: 48–62.

Rodrigues, J., Trombert-Paviot, B., Baud, R., Wagner, J. & Meusnier-Carriot, F. (1997). Galen-in-use : Using artificial intelligence terminology tools to improve the linguistic coherence of a national coding system for surgical procedures, *Proceedings of the 15th International Congress of the European Federation for Medical Informatics, MIE-97*, p. 897Û901.

Rosse, C. & Mejino, J. (2003). A reference ontology for biomedical informatics: the Foundational Model of Anatomy, *Journal of Biomedical Informatics* 36: 478–500.

Sakji, S., Lethord, C., Pereira, S., Dahamna, B., Joubert, M. & Darmoni, S. J. (2009). Drug information portal in Europe: Informatio retrieval with multiple health terminologies, *Stud Health Technol Inform*, Vol. 150, pp. 497–501.

Salton, G. & McGill, M. J. (1983). *Introduction to Modern Information Retrieval*, McGraw-Hill, New York.

Sarker, I., Cantor, M., Gelman, R., Hartel, F. & Lussier, Y. (2003). Linking biomedical language information and knowledge ressources in the 21st Century: GO and UMLS, *Pacific Symposium on BioComputing*, Vol. 8, pp. 439–450.

Shvaiko, P. & Euzenat, J. (2005). A survey of schema-based matching approaches, *Journal on Data Semantics IV* pp. 146–171.

Soualmia, L. (2004). *Towards an intelligent IR through the evaluation of multiple knowledge-based methods of query expansion: application to the health domain on the Internet*, PhD thesis, INSA Roue.

Soualmia, L. F., Griffon, N., Grosjean, J. & Darmoni, S. J. (2011). Improving Information Retrieval by Meta-modelling Medical Terminologies, *Proceedings of 13th Conference on Artificial Intelligence in MEdicine, AIME*, Vol. 6747 of *Lectures Notes in Computer Science*, Springer, pp. 215–219.

Stoilos, G., Stamou, G. & Kollias, S. (2005). A string metric for ontology alignement, *International Semantic Web Conference*, Vol. 3729, pp. 624–637.

Wang, Y., Patrick, J., Miller, G. & O'Hallaran, J. (2008). A computational linguistics motivated mapping of ICPC-2 PLUS to SNOMED CT, *BMC Med Inform Decis Mak* 8 Suppl 1: 5.

Wu, Z. & Palmer, M. (1994). Verb semantics and lexical selection, *32nd Annual Meetings of the Associations for Computational Linguistics*, pp. 133–138.

Zeng, M. & Chan, L. (2004). Trends and issues in establishing interoperability among knowledge organization systems, *Journal of the American Society for Information* 55: 377–395.

Part 3

Clinical Applications

5

Real Time Clinical Decision Support System

Hsueh-Chun Lin
Department of Health Risk Management,
School of Public Health, China Medical University, Taichung,
Taiwan

1. Introduction

Information technology (IT) and Web-based facility have become the major backbone of the modern hospital information systems (HIS) since the beginning of 21st century. Associated with the rapid evolution of medical informatics, the clinical decision support system (CDSS) is playing an important role to help physicians and other healthcare professionals in making decisions while determining diagnosis of patient data. For the routine treatment procedure, the physicians usually take much time to study patients' clinical records (PCRs) prior to explain abstruse clinical markers to patients in clinics. Particularly, for chronic and traceable diseases, they also need to refer patients' quality of life (QOL) and their patient-reported outcomes (PROs) for prescribing the proper therapies. Therefore, a real time clinical decision support system (RTCDSS) is proposed for patient- and clinician-oriented interface as well as patient-to-clinician (P2C) communication, mostly for the chronic diseases with traceable clinical markers. The system provides accurate medical informatics with efficient process for presenting immediately analytical diagram through graphical interface based on patients' and clinicians' requirements.

The major cancer therapy usually brings numbers of side effect in addition to destroy tumors. It implies that QOL is deeply impacted by uncertainty and after-effect due to treatment of oncology clinic. Healthcare people probably make incorrect judgments because patients embarrass on answering private questions or hiding actual conditions. The past studies showed improvements for drug dosing, preventive care, and other economic aspects of medical care, but not convincingly for diagnosis, as reviewing computer-based CDSS on clinician performance and patient outcome (Johnston et al., 1994; Hunt et al., 1998). Obviously, it is not easy to create a universal system for varied clinical requirements. However, it would be possible to build up a platform with expandable components for specified clinical purpose due to customized rules. Therefore, the proposed RTCDSS can be induced by developing a patient-oriented interface with healthcare function to collect real time PROs and PCRs according to practical requirements of hospitals. For example, the assessment of QOL utilizes questionnaires provided by the EORTC[1] to highlight physicians' awareness of patients' status and greatly facilitate physician-patient communication (Detmar et al., 2002). Recently, an interactive assessment system named clinical infometrics

---

[1] European Organization for Research and Treatment of Cancer

was established with information and psychometrics technology for measurement, statistical modeling, informatics and practice, in palliative care with computerized procedure to improve clinical assessment (Chang et al., 2007; Chang, 2008). Applied for measurement and management of PROs, infometrics technique can assist clinicians to more precisely recognize actual response of patients and improve the quality of care with instant process and real time outcomes statistics (Lin et al., 2010). With graphical diagrams, clinicians thus can convince patients by presenting PRO instantly with other PCR.

In clinical practice, furthermore, clinicians meet a number of common problems when it comes to improving quality of clinical treatments as follows: (1) clinicians may take several hours, or even a couple of days, to review PCRs but only have a few minutes to explain their opinions to patients; (2) patients typically find difficulty to understand their condition since clinicians may only explain the disease adequately using written descriptions; (3) the CDSS is computerized, but it may not have online capability in many clinics; (4) real-time analysis is not supported by many commercial computational tools. From clinical data tracking to real-time decision making tools, the flexible Web-based CDSS with online evidence-based medicine (EBM) progress is a growing trend in advanced clinical care The past research indicated that publicly released clinical evidence data assist to improve patient care quality at the hospital level (Fung et al., 2008). Numerous CDSS platforms have been constructed for a variety of clinical approaches. To facilitate the treatments, many studies suggested analytical tools to assist clinicians in estimating the relative pretreatment parameters and for tracking the proper diagnostic guidelines on visualized interfaces (Holmes-Rovner et al., 2005; Walter & Covinsky, 2001; Dorfman et al., 2010). Thus, a clinician-oriented interface with real-time online analysis may improve accuracy and efficiency of decision support. Many clinicians hence are in need of an expandable RTCDSS with an interactive diagrammed interface to efficiently evaluate instant informatics and to make clinical decisions (Lin et al., 2011). It is feasible to take chronic diseases with traceable markers as the case study of RTCDSS.

In order to solidify real time functions of the proposed system, the clinical guideline with medical evidences is recommended for appropriate treatments. The Web-interfaced process has been developed for graphical guidelines that allow users to traverse the algorithm by flowcharts in an interactive fashion (Liem et al., 1995). The clinical benefits were highlighted by rapid knowledge acquisitions, shareable guideline models, and robust information systems while evaluating its impacts on outcomes (Zielstorff, 1998). Thus the electronic guidelines improved decision quality and physician-patients interaction significantly (Hsu et al., 2005). However, many obstacles were encountered as practicing guidelines for the management of workflow integration would be the most difficult tasks (Maviglia et al., 2003). Obviously, lots of challenges still exist while integrating a new RTCDSS with the PROs, PCRs, CDSS, and interactive guidelines into the legacy HIS. The framework for interactive clinical guidelines should consider readiness of clinicians for practice, barriers to change as experienced by clinicians, and the target level of interventions (Moulding et al., 1999). To properly integrate electronic clinical guidance into an existing system, the issues of heterogeneous data integration should be practiced in the platform. Numerous studies established models of evidence-based guidelines by using XML (extensible mark-up language) documents (Shiffman et al., 2000; Sanders et al., 2001) and AJAX (asynchronous

JavaScript and XML) technique to supply shareable information and user-friendly search, respectively, with automatic completion. The techniques have been widely utilized to online interactive interface in the past years for acquisition of efficient data transportation.

In this article, prostate cancer, which is familiarly monitored by prostate specific antigen (PSA) and other treatment parameters, is taken to practice the proposed RTCDSS. A Web-based platform is established with clinical infometrics and interactive guidelines for a RTCDSS. Java™ technologies are applied to create patient- and clinician-oriented interfaces with automatic clinical procedure and data transformation.

2. Development of RTCDSS infrastructure

This section will describe the details how the Web-based platform of RTCDSS is built upon novel Internet technologies. The infrastructure involves core models as follows: model view controller (MVC), object oriented mapping (ORM), clinical data warehouse (CDW), Web services (WS), online analytical process (OLAP), and AJAX. Data flows throughout all stages of the structure can be manipulated by Internet services and information techniques.

2.1 Model-view-controller model

The MVC model is a type of design patterns employed in software engineering. It hybridizes the design patterns, and divides system responsibilities into three parts: the model, which maintains program data and logic; the view, which provides a visual presentation of the model; the controller, which processes user input and makes modifications to the model. Herein, it is utilized for generating a modelized architecture systematically with expandable and reusable components of the Web-based platform for efficient and flexible collaboration. The concept of modelized architecture can be driven into Web assessment for acquiring PROs from online infometrics system and adapting PCRs with the legacy HIS in hospital. The architecture reflects the MVC design pattern, which was established in 1970′ and included several design patterns to build reliable object-oriented software system (Krasner & Pope, 1988). The public of design patterns was first made by introducing twenty-three patterns related to creational, structural and behavioural models for software design to progress recurrent elements (Gamma et al., 1994). The MVC theoretically hybrids three of them, the "strategy," "observer," and "composite" patterns; and divides system responsibilities into the model, the view, and the controller. The pattern is involved in well-known open-source framework such as "Strut," "Spring," "Hibernate" for development. These frameworks with MVC paradigm use polling for its input control to solve the problems on consuming computation resources when the user is not interacting with the interface and avoid unnecessary performance loss. Due to this architecture, a web-based prototype system built with the open-source framework is available for online infometrics of QOL. Fig 1 presents an architecture consisting of conceptual components organized by three main groups which contain the model, the view, and the controller to provide sole modules but support one another for system requirements.

As extending the MVC-based architecture to the RTCDSS, the built-in elements within the framework should be reusable and extractable to enable clinical analysis and decision support for clinical cares which includes: (a) instantaneous disease evaluation, (b) risk analysis, and (c) treatment guidance. For these tasks, the infrastructure can be detailed below to complete requests for presentation, management, analysis, and database.

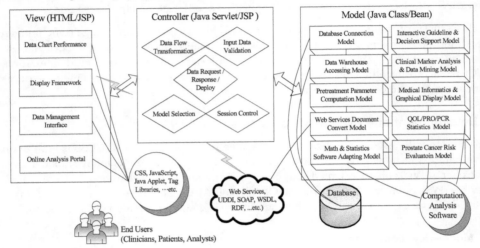

Fig. 1. Web MVC-based Architecture with model-view-controller components.

i.   Models:

The models are leading four main groups: disease evaluation, risk analysis, treatment guidance, and data processing models. The first three models are relative to clinical data computation while the last one represents the other IT modules. The disease evaluation contains modules primarily to retrieve clinical variables, calculate pretreatment parameters, and evaluate PROs and PCRs. The risk analysis model drives algorithms to analyze clinical variables and parameters, identify risk indicators and criteria, and so on. The guidance criteria model enables the generation of evidence-based diagrams, online guidance and decision support. The rest of the IT-related modules such as clinical data conversion, database connection, and graphical display, are included in the data processing model.

ii. Views:

The views can implement the patient- and clinician-oriented interfaces directly with the OLAP portal and the EBM informatics for clinicians at the presentation stage. Similarly, the view of management interface provides IT engineers with security administration at the management stage. Meanwhile, all clinical data can be taken care through the analysis view at the analysis and database stages. Based on this consideration, these views are behind the major components of each stage such as real-time diagrams, interactive guidelines, privilege administration, informatics management, data filtering and data analysis tools.

iii. Controllers:

The controllers support interactions among the models and views within the RTCDSS infrastructure. At the presentation stage, the controllers process data flow transformation and data input validation when the clinicians begin online inquiries. At the management stage, the privilege control and role identification are required when the engineers are conducting system maintenance. Meanwhile, the clinical data at the back stages of analysis and database are coordinated by heterogeneous data transaction.

2.2 Object relation mapping model

Object-relational mapping (ORM) is a programming technique to convert data between incompatible type systems in relational databases and object-oriented languages. It is the automated and transparent persistence of application objects to the tables in a relational database by using metadata that describes the mapping between the objects and the database. The ORM works through reversibly transforming data from one representation to another and is used to unify various data format transformed among the sub systems (Bauger & King, 2005). We can coordinate the infometrics and clinical data flow through the interface of ORM to convert persistent objects and manage data transaction and resource throughout database. The interface includes functional modules of session, session factory, configuration, transaction, query, and criteria to interact XML metadata with application modules of server. In mechanism, the session interface conducts lightweight instances of application in safe as the necessary data are requested on the web tier all the time; the application obtains session instances from a session factory to share many application modules and cache scripted database transaction and other mapping metadata at runtime for data conversion. Then, the configuration interface configures the location of mapping documents and specific properties for data retrieval; thus a transaction interface is optionally selected to keep portable between different execution environments. Furthermore, the query interface performs instances to control data queries against the database, while the criteria interface executes queries under the objected-oriented criterion. Herein, the assessment of QOL questionnaires can be implemented by the ORM model for online analysis to concurrently process and share light weight data over the Web-based system by rearranging storage, organization, and retrieval of structured data.

2.3 Clinical data warehouse model

The data warehouse is known as an integral database for historical data repository with lack of systematic arrangement by information technique. It was initially defined as an integrated, subject-oriented, time-variant and non-volatile database that provides support for decision making (Inmon & Kelley, 1994). The concept of clinical data warehouse obeys the definition above to integrate practical PROs and PCRs with a standard procedure from different hospital databases into the knowledge bank for advanced analysis. To incorporate infometrix data with existing PCR for online analysis, a clinical data warehouse (CDW) is planned and practiced in the RTCDSS. The data warehouse is known as building up an integral database for historical data repository with lack of systematic arrangement by information technique. The critical factor leading to the use of data warehouse is that a data analyst can perform complex queries and analyses without slowing down the operating system. The raw data for clinic in variety of format would be rigorously unified by extract-transform-load (ETL) process into database through extraction, consolidation, filtering, transformation, cleansing, conversion and aggregation (Rob & Cornel, 2004). As planning the data warehouse, fact tables and cube dimensions related to historical data are the key elements. The fact table contains facts that are linked through their dimensions, which are qualifying characteristics that provide additional perspectives to the given facts.

2.4 Web services model

A Web service is an interface describing a collection of operations that are network accessible through standardized XML messaging (Gottschalk et al., 2002). With the Web services model, the criterion for decision support can be retrieved from online data logs for online analysis. Through Web services, the computation model retrieved decision criteria from unified document to create online statistical chart. In order to improve efficiency of data transaction, the intensive database query is executed to remain at the server site and the less-intensive data for online analysis is processed at the client site. The designation of XML schema is the essential factor of Web services for accessing network data. The tree structure with hieratical node elements is created in the document of XML schema to record data from the web server, and then the XML parser can parse the tree structure by subsequent nodes in the schema to retrieve data. The flow chart of parsing process in Fig 2 is separated as three parts: (1) converse data as XML document from database based on the specific schema, (2) parse XML document through SAX (Simple Application-programming-interface for XML) standard, and (3) retrieve data of XML document by scheme definition. The interactive data required by QOL assessment and guideline conduction are then transformed as Web services documents. The historical clinical data redeemed by expert opinions will feedback to data warehouse; and, the online computation models retrieve decision criteria from unified documents to display statistical charts. Herein, the WS model is integrated with the ORM model to share the QOL questionnaires as the over the Web-based system for indexing and reorganizing the clinical database.

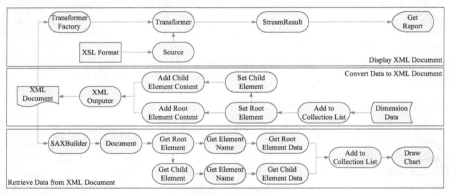

Fig. 2. Parsing procedure for light-weight data with XML schema.

2.5 Online analytical process model

Online analytical process (OLAP) has been embedded on the decision support platform deployed for enterprise system since early period of network boom-up era (Chaudhuri & Dayal, 1997). It provides efficient functionalities with computation algorithm on data warehouse to explore historical data. This model can help in presenting real time analytical information by online graphical diagraph with specific computation modules. In order to manage and analyze infometrix and clinical data cooperatively in the system, the OLAP model crossing over the web server and database leads online computation within the RTCDSS. The PCR queries integrated with heterogeneous databases are primarily progressed while accessing the database server; thus, the risk evaluations embedded within online session logs are efficiently retrieved as connecting the web server. The progress may keep complex query behind data mining for the knowledge bank but remain simple data transaction through dynamic views in data warehouse. Based on the MVC architecture, the online clinical informatics can be achieved by the OLAP mechanism. For example, the clinician is a decision maker on a presentation stage that performs the components of the interactive guideline and real-time diagrams in clinic.

2.6 Asynchronous JavaScript XML-HttpRequest model

The asynchronous JavaScript XML-HttpRequest (AJAX) technique has been widely applied for online interactive interface in the past years to grab instant information as well as to avoid lag in transportation of client-server data. It can be developed as diverse, convenient, and interactive applications with visualized functions for user-friendly interface design. The basic concept of asynchronous data transformation is storing transient data at client sites to reduce redundant data query with database sites and enhance interactive patient- and clinician-oriented interface. Adaptive with the client-server network architecture, it may process numerous data queries between the database and the web server. Technically, persistent and large data transaction might downgrade the network speed. As the WS and OLAP models communicate with the client browser for adopting light-weight data like QOL questionnaires, risk evaluations or guideline indexes, the AJAX model helps in adjusting data interaction performance. The method doesn't need to request database all the time but load into browser's temporary container at client site. If the client site keeps sessions at online status, the browser is calling JavaScript™ and restoring data. Once the session needs reconnection or updating, the client-server communication is activating. The manner can be approved by AJAX that is a standards-based programming technique to make web-based applications more responsive, interactive, and customizable in addition to reduce network latency and interface complexity for keeping server responsiveness (Smith, 2006).

In short, the proposed RTCDSS remains heavy-weight database query at server site and keeps light-weight data for online analysis at client site to improve clinical data transaction efficiently. In the system, clinical data are analyzed to yield expert opinions for feedback to clinical data warehouse. Through models of ORM, WS and OLAP, the decision criteria and interactive guidance are displayed by AJAX with real time online diagraphs. Based on the MVC and CDW, the web and database servers are collaborative within the network services.

3. Design of patient and clinician oriented interfaces

This section aims to integrate previous models with practical clinical interfaces for both of patients and clinicians. In which, prostate cancer is selected for the sample of modeling since it is the chronic disease with a traceable marker for long-term monitoring. Two types of interfaces are addressed below for processing PRO with clinical infometrics and analyzing PCRs upon the EBM. The entire infrastructure is designed with five primary layers to (1) acquire patient-reported outcomes at the "acquisition", (2) present online clinical diagraph at the "presentation", (3) manage clinical information at the "management", (4) analyze patient's clinical records at the "analysis", and (5) coalesce diverse clinical databases at the "database". The structure is exampled by the project named clinical infometrics for prostate cancer (CIPC) in China Medical University Hospital (CMUH) in Tahchung, Taiwan.

3.1 Patient-oriented interface

The ORM and CDW models are driven for the patient-oriented interface to collaborate clinical measurements with medical informatics through Internet. A knowledge bank is generated in database with feedback of expert opinions that provide clinicians real time guidance. Instant assessment of patients' QOL is acquired to compare with clinical markers.

3.1.1 QOL assessment

Herein, an infometrics system upon real time online assessment is developed for prostate cancer patients. It is employed by the RTCDSS to generate psychometrical modules upon information technique to measure patient's QOL. The assessment results can be instantly reported while patients are conducted to easily complete questionnaires on the interface of patient-oriented design. Compared to importance of survival evaluation, QOL becomes a significant index of healthcare. EORTC creates series of QOL assessments in cancer clinical trials to provide a more accurate evaluation of the well-being of individuals or groups of patients and of the benefits and side-effects that may result from medical intervention. The reliability, validity and sensitivity of assessment are acceptable since questionnaires have been validated by more than 3,000 studies worldwide. The quality of life questionnaire (QLQ) C30 is developed to assess the QOL of cancer patients while the PR25 is designed for prostate cancer patients. In the CIPC, a web-based platform with infometrics system is to serve prostate cancer patients. The questionnaires are adopted from EORTC, thus QLQ C30 and PR25 are the primary assessment modules for volunteer patients in pilot study. The C30 involves 9 multi-item scales for 5 functional scales (physical, role, cognitive, emotional, and social), 3 symptom scales (fatigue, pain, and nausea and vomiting), and 1 global health QOL scale, while several single-item symptom measures are also included (Aaronson, N.K., et al., 1993). The PR25 is a 25-item questionnaire for use among patients with localized and metastatic prostate cancer. It has subscales assessing urinary symptoms (9 items), bowel symptoms (4 items), treatment-related symptoms (6 items) and sexual functioning (6 items).

3.1.2 Clinical implementation for prostate cancer

QOL is an important healthcare index but patients probably conceal the truth because of private manners. In addition, the traditional paper-based QOL assessment usually causes reading difficulty for patients because of improper font size and print space. Hence the infometrics module of CIPC system is designed for patient orientation through sufficient accessibility and accompanies QLQ with instant PRO analysis and evaluation. In which, the fonts of questionnaires are enlarged for elderly patients who have poor eyesight and the selection buttons are displayed on a touch screen for patients who are not familiar with using computer mouse. Most of prostate caner patients are seniors who initially might not know how to click mouse-button or scroll the browser to navigate the computer; therefore the Web-page design is simplified by one-touch action per question before the users are well trained. Besides, a multimedia function played with head phones is optionally provided for low education level patients who could read questions with limited literacy. Patients are arranged privately in a consulting room to complete the questionnaires while waiting for the clinicians. Then, through automatic computation and statistical models, the clinicians could immediately evaluate the real time reports with online analysis. Based on the system design, clinicians and researchers can immediately access infometrix data after patients completed the questionnaires. Fig 3 performs the operating procedure, in which the clinician can make cross compare overall treatment information with instant expert opinions for advanced communicate with patients.

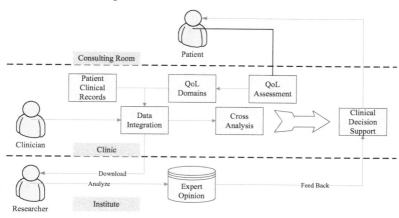

Fig. 3. Clinic progress implemented with clinical infometrics system.

Furthermore, the network of CIPC needs to link hospital and campus networks, but under hospital's information security policy, to collaborate tiers of database, analysis, management, presentation, and acquisition for clinical and research workflows. As shown in Fig 4, the database tier supports clinical and infometrix data warehouse; the analysis tier assists analysts analyzing data and feeds back statistical results as resource of the

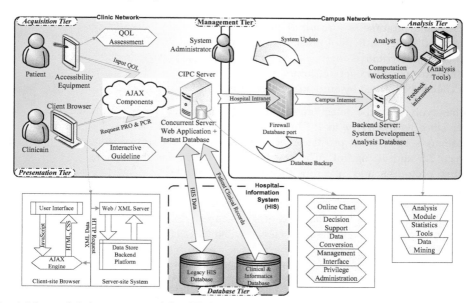

Fig. 4. Network infrastructure of the CIPC system with RTCDSS components.

knowledge bank; the management tier is the control center for administrating data flow throughout the entire system; the presentation tier presents real-time functions for online decision support and interactive guideline on a friendly interface for P2C communication; the acquisition tier becomes the data collector to execute online QOL assessment with accessibility interface. The infrastructure bridges both networks of clinics and campus through the firewall to routinely backup clinical data and maintain the CIPC system.

3.2 Clinician-oriented interface

The clinician-oriented interface is established by MVC model to help analyzing pretreatment parameters for clinical evidences. The system can be constructed by the open source frameworks with the graphical diagrams to combine PCRs and biomarkers from diverse database through networks. In the CIPC, the interface can guide clinicians to concurrently collect and analyze specific clinical markers with instant diagrams for prostate cancer patients. By referring suggestions from participant clinicians for long-term tracking, we herein create computation models based on statistical algorithms to respond expert opinions.

3.2.1 Prostate cancer treatment

Several pretreatment parameters and clinical markers are significant for tracking the disease condition of prostate cancer patients periodically. The CIPC system is proposed in urology clinic for reflecting relationship between QOL and pretreatment parameters such as PSA, clinical classification stage, and Gleason score, etc. Prostate cancer rarely causes symptoms early in the course of the disease. Suspicion of prostate cancer resulting in prostatic biopsy is most often raised by abnormalities found on digital rectal examination (DRE). The presence of systemic symptoms as a result of prostate cancer suggests locally advanced or widely metastatic disease. Growth of prostate cancer into the urethra or bladder neck can result in obstructive and irritative voiding symptoms (Carter et al., 2007). Prostate cancer has greatly benefited from the discovery of tumor markers. Instant observation and comparison of PRO and PCR can be tracked by auto-analysis prior to clinics.

PSA has evolved for the detection, staging, and monitoring of men diagnosed with prostate cancer since its discovery in 1979 to clinical application in the late 1980s through 1990s (Sensabaugh, 1978). Most prostate cancer arises as clinically nonpalpable disease with PSA between 2.5 and 10 ng/mL. The stage regarding how far the tumors have spread for defining prognosis and selecting therapies, and has become an important marker as evaluating prostate cancer. The four-stage TNM system, which includes the size of the tumor (T), the number of involved lymph nodes (N), and the presence of any other metastases (M), indicate how far the cancer has spread for defining prognosis and selecting therapies. Among urologic malignancies, the combination of DRE and serum PSA is the most useful first-line test for assessing the risk of prostate cancer. Particularly, the initial PSA value after a treatment is the most useful clinical information for detecting, staging, and monitoring prostate cancer patients when assessing the risk of prostate cancer (Partin et al., 1997; Pound et al., 1999). The clinical variables can be retrieved from databases of HIS through different networks.

i.   PSA Level

The presence of prostate diseases is the most important factor affecting serum levels of PSA (Wang et al., 1981; Ercole et al., 1987). Many studies have made efforts to evaluate other thresholds to maximize the positive biopsy rate of PSA-based screening (Gann et al., 1995). The PSA-related parameters including PSA density (PSAD), PSA velocity (PSAV) and PSA doubling time (PSADT) are considered to improve diagnostic accuracy of PSA. A direct relationship between PSAD and the likelihood of cancer has been documented (Bazinet et al., 1994), and higher PSA densities may be found among groups of men with positive biopsies compared with men with negative biopsies (Uzzo et al., 1995). PCRs can be filtered to rank high risk patients who have relatively smaller prostate volumes when a constant number of biopsies are obtained.

PSAV is the rate of change in serum PSA. A rate in excess of 0.75 ng/mL per year is a significant indicator of prostate cancer for prediction of prostate cancer (Carter et al., 1992; D'Amico et al., 2005). PSAV can be estimated by substituting PSA data into the linear regression equation as Eq.(1) that formulates the arbitrary PSA (P_i) with respect to time (T_i).

$$P_i = \alpha + \beta \times T_i \tag{1}$$

Where, the parameter β represents the slope of equation and is identical to the PSAV while α would be the initial PSA. T_i is available to count by days, months or years.

PSADT is denoted as the duration when the logarithm of PSA doubles and has been evaluated in patients with a rising PSA after local treatment with radiation therapy (Fowler et al., 1994). In Eq. (2), we can substitute the regression equation of PSAV into the half-logarithmic coordinate of $\ln(P_i)$ versus T_i, and a straight line is obtained to calculate doubling PSA at doubling time T_D.

$$\frac{\ln(2 \times P_1) - \ln(P_1)}{T_D - T_1} = \frac{\ln(P_2) - \ln(P_1)}{T_2 - T_1} \text{ yields } T_D - T_1 = \frac{\ln(2) \times (T_2 - T_1)}{\ln(P_2) - \ln(P_1)} \tag{2}$$

The relationship of two arbitrary PSAs measured at the time T_1 and T_2 with respect to the doubling time T_D is formulated when $\ln(2*P_1)$ is estimated.

ii.   TNM stage

The well-known TNM classification system generally evaluates the size of the tumor (T) by four stages, the extent of involved lymph nodes (N) by two stages, and any metastasis (M) by two stages. For evaluation of the primary tumor: T1 stage presents tumor, but not detectable clinically or with imaging; in T2, the tumor can be palpated on examination, but has not spread outside the prostate; the tumor has spread through the prostatic capsule in T3 stage; and in T4, the tumor has invaded other nearby structures. For evaluation of the regional lymph nodes: N0 present there has been no spread to the regional lymph nodes whereas N1 has been spread. For evaluation of distance metastasis, M0 represent there is no distant metastasis while M1 has that. In this study, version 6 of the TNM system published by the American Joint Committee for Cancer (AJCC) and the International Union against Cancer (UICC) in 2002 is adopted.

iii.   Gleason score

The Gleason grading system is based on a low-magnification microscopic description of the architecture of the cancer and is the most commonly used classification scheme for the histological grading of prostate cancer (Gleason, 1966). The predominant pattern that occupies the largest area of the specimen is given a grade between 1 and 5. This number is then added to the grade assigned to the second most dominant pattern; thus, a Gleason sum can be arranged between 2 and 10. This system describes tumors as "well", "moderately", and "poorly" differentiated based on Gleason score of 2-4, 5-6, and 7-10, respectively.

iv.   Kaplan Meier survival estimation

The Kaplan-Meier estimator, which is known as the product limit estimator, estimates the survival function from life-time data (Kaplan & Meier, 1958). Let S(t) be the probability that an item from a given group of size N will have a lifetime exceeding t. Corresponding to each t_i is n_i, the number "at risk" just prior to time t_i, and d_i, the number of deaths at time t_i, where i = 1, 2, ..., N. Note that t_i is equal or less than t_{i+1} and the intervals between each time typically will not be uniform. Then, the estimator is with nonparametric maximum likelihood convergence of S(t) in a product of the form

$$S(t) = \prod_{t_i < t} \frac{n_i - d_i}{n_i} \tag{3}$$

When there is no censoring, n_i is the number of survivors just prior to time t_i. With censoring, n_i is the number of survivors less the number of losses. It is only those surviving cases that are still being observed that are "at risk" of an observed death.

v.   Cox Proportional Hazard Model

Proportional hazards model is a sub-class of survival models well known in statistics by consisting of two parts: the underlying hazard function to describe how hazard (risk) changes over time; and the effect parameters to describe how hazard relates to other factors, e.g. the choice of treatment, in a typical medical example. The effect parameters estimated by any proportional hazards model can be reported as hazard ratios. The formula in Eq. (4) is recruited for building computation module in the system.

$$h(t, \mathbf{X}) = h_0(t) \exp(\sum_{i=1}^{p} \beta_i X_i), \quad X = (X_1, X_2, \cdots X_p) \tag{4}$$

In which, $h_0(t)$ is the baseline hazard involving t but not X's while X denotes a collection of p explanatory variables X_1, X_2, ..., X_p and the model is nonparametric because $h_0(t)$ is unspecified. For PSA variables correlation in prostate cancer treatment, these variables may include age, race, initial PSA, PSAV, PSAD, clinical stage, treatment, and so on.

3.2.2 Instant analytical diagram

The computation models involve statistical modules to achieve pretreatment parameters for clinical requirements. These modules carry out analytical diagrams on the clinician-oriented interface for physicians to instantly study tendency of illness conditions according to the significant pretreatment parameters below.

i. PSA-related information

The PSA-related information such as PSAD, PSAV and PSADT can be calculated due to previous equations and perform real time online analytical diagrams. The graphic interface displays instant diagram of PSA baseline with respect to parameters above. The clinicians can select required item to present possible velocity and doubling time of PSA by checking the date of PSA record from check-box. The diagram can be printed out as the attachment of clinical prescription. Furthermore, the survival and hazard estimation modules are available for instant crossing comparison to avoid time-consuming manual analysis beyond clinics.

ii. Partin table

Gleason grade has been shown to correlate with the pathologic extent of disease but is not sufficiently accurate so that Partin tables are usually referred. The Partin tables include primary clinical stage, serum PSA level, and Gleason score to determine the probability of having a final pathologic stage based on logistic regression analyses for all 3 variables combined (Partin et al., 1993; Partin et al., 2001). The table is important in guiding decisions for prostate cancer. It is a way of predicting cancer's pathologic stage which is determined after the prostate gland has been surgically removed and examined by a pathologist. The probability is referred by following the pathologic stages, due to the tables, as (1) organ-confined disease, (2) established capsular penetration, (3) seminal vesicle involvement, and (4) lymph node involvement. If probability of organ-confined disease is high, then early-stage treatment options are feasible. If the probability of cancer having spread beyond the prostate is high, then other treatment options will need to be considered. Herein, the system adopts the Partin table guided by the National Comprehensive Cancer Network (NCCN).

iii. Risk evaluation criteria

Risk evaluation criteria of prostate cancer is constructed on the basis of large numbers of patients who have undergone radical prostatectomy to aid in the precise prediction of pathologic stage by using multiple clinical parameters as accurate predictors of both cancer extent and long-term outcomes after treatment of the primary tumor (Kleer & Oesterling, 1993). The criteria as shown in Table 1 (D'Amico et al., 2001) can be adopted to stratify patients into low, intermediate, and high risk disease, and to summarize the failure status,

Risk group	Risk factors	Risk (a, b, c) %
Low	T1c or T2a and PSA <= 10 ng/ml and Gleason score <= 6	(<25, 85, 83)
Intermediate	T2b or Gleason score = 7 or PSA > 10 and <= 20 ng/ml	(25-50, 60, 46)
High	T2c or PSA > 20 ng/ml or Gleason score >= 8	(>50, 30, 29)
a. Post-therapy PSA failure at 5 yrs; b. PSA failure-free survival at 5 yrs; c. PSA failure-free survival at 10 yrs		

Table 1. Risk Evaluations for Prostate Cancer (D'Amico et al., 2001; Lin et al., 2011).

Based on the correlations of these pretreatment parameters with the true extent of disease, the RTCDSS can integrate the clinical data and expert opinions available for clinicians to determine the likelihood of disease progression and predict the pathologic stage.

3.3 Integration design

Based on RTCDSS design, the CIPC system is built with open source framework of Java™ technique while Apache Tomcat™ and Oracle™ are selected as Web and database servers, respectively. The system components with flexible functionality and keep-in-simple-stupid (KISS) interface are designed to enhance the human computer interaction. The system involves database, analysis, management, presentation, and acquisition layers, from right to left in Fig 5, on the modelized architecture by implementing previous methodology.

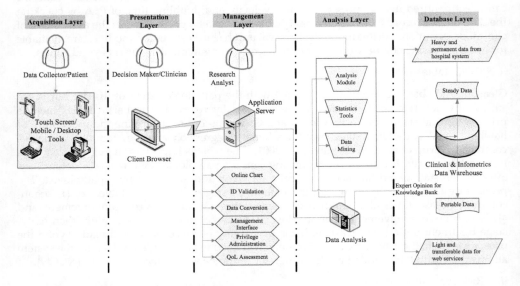

Fig. 5. Five-layer development of RTCDSS infrastructure (Lin et al., 2010).

1. The database layer is the foundation of the system for building clinical data warehouse. Fig 6 illustrates the primary object relationship diagram and schema simplified by entity relationship diagram (ERD), where the attributes denote correlation between QOL domains and treatment effects. The schema combined two sets of fact tables for infometrix and clinical records so that "Answer_Full" and "Answer_Domain" tables store and transform assessment data to QOL domain score, while "Patient_Info" and "Prostate_Cancer" tables retrieve data from PCR. "Answer_Index" is an index table to bridge "Answer" and "Question" tables, which request and arrange assessment data, and derive cube dimensions of PSA, treatment, clinical stages and Gleason scores.

2. The analysis layer assists researchers analyzing data and feeds back statistical results as resource of knowledge bank. In the practice, several types of data file formats converted from database were generated to satisfy different progresses supported by analysis tools. The layer incorporates database and application servers with remote computation or offline data mining and feed expert opinions back to knowledge bank of RTCDSS.

3. The management layer plays the role of control center for managing data flow within the entire system. A management interface is designed to enhance capability of data access functions for health care people and researchers to plot online charts, identify single sign-on, process data conversion, administrate user privilege, and acquire QOL assessment. All modules are built as objects of models for sharing functionality but secured with privilege roles of health care people, clinicians and researchers.

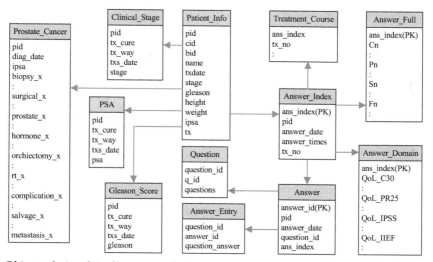

Fig. 6. Object relationship diagram and schema (Lin et al., 2010).

4. The presentation layer is the interface of real time decision support for communication of patients and clinicians. The system presented instantaneous statistical diagrams by referencing expert opinions from knowledge bank for clinicians. In the CIPC, it performs the real time QOL evaluation with respect to mean value of other patients, initial PSA, Gleason score, treatment stage, etc. Clinicians are able to indicate treatment indexes online through graphical interface for decision support.

5. The acquisition layer becomes the data receiver of the system to execute QLQ online behind accessibility interface design. Perhaps most of patients fell uncomfortable, either in physical or mental status, and avoid writing paper sheet by themselves as answering the assessment questions. In the practice, the touched screen, the sizeable large fonts, and the audio media with ear phones are functioned for more accessibilities of patients.

Based on the system design, clinicians and researchers are available to access infometrix data after patients finished assessments through patient-oriented interface. For securing patients' privacy, the clinical records must be forbidden from internet users except of particular clinical people; therefore, the primary database server for instant infometrix becomes the data center in clinic site; meanwhile, a backup database server in research site allows restore data automatically through specified protocol.

4. Practice of patient-to-clinician strategy

The mechanism of innovative CIPC is compiled with online assessments of QOL and PRO modules and the interactive interface is functioned for clinical requirement to efficiently automate the clinical procedure. Beyond the patient- and clinician- oriented interfaces, the P2C communication becomes the strategy through interactive guideline with treatment risk evaluation to provide real time references for decision making. For adapting the CIPC with the P2C strategy into hospital, quasi-real time data transportation is adopted for flexibly arranging administration schedules due to the hospital management policy.

4.1 Interactive guideline

The proposed framework was practiced in the urological cancer department of CMUH. Both of the campus and hospital networks were incorporated with heterogeneous database management. The necessary prostate cancer data resources were extracted and filtered from the cancer data center of CMUH. The interactive guidance design for clinician-oriented interface is evaluated with regard to how well it helps clinicians interact with patients and provide efficient clinical care. With practice of the CIPC system, PROs with QOL can be collected through clinical infometrics and be referred by interactive guidelines for clinical decision support. Herein, the guideline with QOL domains, risk evaluation table, interactive treatment chart, and automated prescription will be discussed. Through the RTCDSS, the approaches regarding clinical infometrics for patient outcome collection of QOL and interactive guideline for clinical decision support will be highlighted below.

i.   Statistics of QOL domains – The diagram on Fig 7 lists details of the last assessment results involving the questionnaires, range and scale in each domain, effect and missing items while answering questions. All QOL domains reflect the functions and symptoms of a patient in physical and mental conditions during the treatment cycle. Clinicians can realize statistic results of patient's disease conditions at the beginning of clinic. The historical QOL scores with PSA values shown in Fig 8 provide an overall chart for clinician and patient. It helps the patient describe their real health condition to avoid ambiguous conversation.

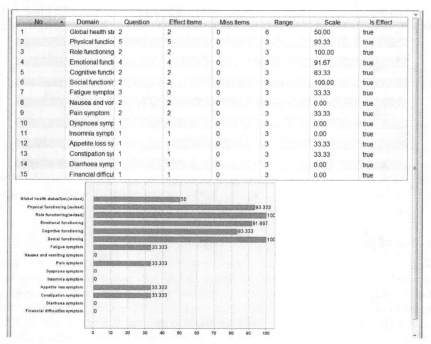

No	Domain	Question	Effect Items	Miss Items	Range	Scale	Is Effect
1	Global health sta	2	2	0	6	50.00	true
2	Physical functior	5	5	0	3	93.33	true
3	Role functioning	2	2	0	3	100.00	true
4	Emotional functi	4	4	0	3	91.67	true
5	Cognitive functic	2	2	0	3	83.33	true
6	Social functionir	2	2	0	3	100.00	true
7	Fatigue symptor	3	3	0	3	33.33	true
8	Nausea and von	2	2	0	3	0.00	true
9	Pain symptom	2	2	0	3	33.33	true
10	Dyspnoea symp	1	1	0	3	0.00	true
11	Insomnia sympt	1	1	0	3	0.00	true
12	Appetite loss sy	1	1	0	3	33.33	true
13	Constipation syr	1	1	0	3	33.33	true
14	Diarrhoea symp	1	1	0	3	0.00	true
15	Financial difficul	1	1	0	3	0.00	true

Fig. 7. Statistics of QOL domains (Lin et al., 2010).

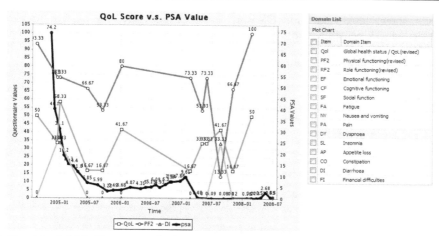

Fig. 8. Graphical QOL diagram with clinical marker - QOL vs. PSA baseline (Lin et al., 2010).

ii. Disease evaluation of the PSA level – Fig. 9 shows the PSAV and PSADT values with PSA baseline while the clinician enters the patient's ID and selects an arbitrary time interval. The real-time diagram shows the disease information of the patient's PSA level throughout different treatments. It can be seen that the system retrieved the patient's data from PCRs and listed related pretreatment parameters for an overview of the patient's disease history. The baseline of PSA is completely plotted during different treatment cycles with significant points (such as the initial PSA) of note.

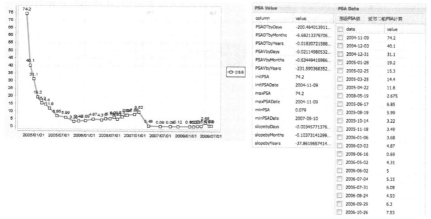

Fig. 9. Interactive guidance to help computing PSA-related data online (Lin et al., 2011).

iii. Risk guidance with the Partin table – Using the Partin table module in the system, the clinician can easily find and input pretreatment parameters such as PSA, Gleason score, and a clinical stage to determine the risk percentage shown in Fig 10. The clinician can find and input pretreatment parameters like PSA, Gleason score and clinical stage for determining the risk percentage. In this case, the clinician input T1c, 32.4, and 5-6 for

TNM stage, PSA value and Gleason grade, respectively; the system immediately estimated risk percentage in high risk group due to Table 1 that shows more than 50% for 5 years of post-therapy PSA failure as well as 30% and 29% for 5-year and 10-year PSA failure-free survival, respectively.

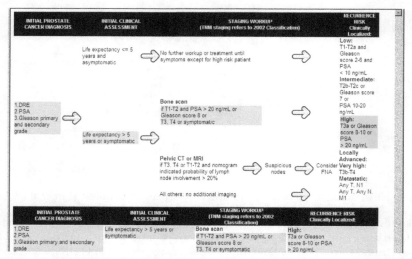

			TABLE I. Clinical Stage T1c (nonpalpable, PSA elevated)				
PSA Range (ng/mL)	Pathologic Stage		Gleason Score				
		2-4	5-6	3+4=7	4+3=7	8-10
0-2.5	Organ confined	95 (89-99)	90 (88-93)	79 (74-85)	71 (62-79)	66 (54-78)
	Extraprostatic extension	5 (1-11)	9 (7-12)	17 (13-23)	25 (18-34)	28 (20-38)
	Seminal vesicle (+)	—	0 (0-1)	2 (1-5)	2 (1-5)	4 (1-10)
	Lymph node (+)	—	—	1 (0-2)	1 (0-4)	1 (0-4)
2.6-4.0	Organ confined	92 (82-98)	84 (81-90)	68 (62-74)	58 (48-67)	52 (41-63)
	Extraprostatic extension	8 (2-18)	15 (13-18)	27 (22-33)	37 (29-46)	40 (31-50)
	Seminal vesicle (+)	—	1 (0-1)	4 (2-7)	4 (1-7)	6 (3-12)
	Lymph node (+)	—	—	1 (0-2)	1 (0-3)	1 (0-4)
4.1-6.0	Organ confined	90 (78-98)	80 (78-83)	63 (58-68)	52 (43-60)	46 (36-56)
	Extraprostatic extension	10 (2-22)	19 (16-21)	32 (27-36)	42 (38-50)	45 (36-54)
	Seminal vesicle (+)	—	1 (0-1)	3 (2-5)	3 (1-6)	6 (3-9)
	Lymph node (+)	—	0 (0-1)	2 (1-3)	3 (1-5)	3 (1-6)
6.1-10.0	Organ confined	87 (73-97)	75 (72-77)	54 (49-59)	43 (35-51)	37 (28-46)
	Extraprostatic extension	13 (3-27)	23 (21-25)	36 (32-40)	47 (40-54)	48 (39-57)
	Seminal vesicle (+)	—	2 (2-3)	5 (5-11)	5 (4-12)	13 (8-19)
	Lymph node (+)	—	0 (0-1)	2 (1-3)	2 (1-4)	3 (1-5)
>10.0	Organ confined	80 (61-95)	62 (58-64)	37 (32-42)	27 (21-34)	22 (15-30)
	Extraprostatic extension	20 (5-38)	33 (30-36)	43 (38-48)	51 (44-58)	50 (42-58)
	Seminal vesicle (+)	—	4 (3-5)	12 (9-17)	11 (6-17)	17 (10-25)
	Lymph node (+)	—	2 (1-3)	8 (5-11)	10 (5-17)	11 (6-18)

Clinical Stage: T1c
PSA Value: 32.4
Gleason Score: 5-6

Submit

Profile :
Clinical Stage   T1c
Gleason Score   5-6
PSA   32.4

Recurrence Risk :
High Risk Group :
5 years of posttherapy PSA failure : >50%
5-year PSA failure-free survival : 30%
10-year PSA failure-free survival : 29%

Pathological Stage :
Organ confined   62(58-64)
Extraprostatic extension 33(30-36)
Seminal vesicle (+)   4(3-5)
Lymph node (+)   2(1-3)

Fig. 10. A screen shot of real-time decision support that the clinician can use to evaluate the recurrence risk and the Partin table online by flexibly adjusting clinical data (Lin et al., 2011).

iv. Interactive guidelines for treatment reference – Clinicians can interact with the guideline thus the phase of treatment procedure based on the criteria are carried out for decision making as PCRs are input. For example on Fig 11, if the PSA was 25.5ng/ml, the clinical stage was T3, Gleason score was 8, life expectancy was more than 5 years,

Fig. 11. Interactive guideline of CIPC system for overview guidance that can highlight a suitable prostate cancer treatment flow based on a patient's clinical data.

with symptomatic therapy as bone scan; the blue region will pop up for overview and be duplicated to the bottom area of the screen to signify the cure steps for reference. Meanwhile, the risk evaluation will be highlighted by yellow mark at the right side. By providing a comparison with the non-highlighted steps on the overview of guideline flow, the flowchart allows the clinicians to identify the current stage and see what the next step is.

v. Special diagnostic chart for automated prescription – To prevent typing error by clinicians as input electronic PCRs, the design of special diagnostic chart lists primary clinical markers for selection. Fig 12 displays an interface that the clinician can select required item to immediately produce unified statement of automated prescription as concurrently inputting data into the database for related hospital information systems.

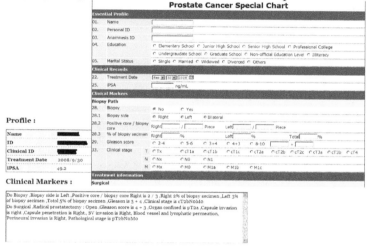

Fig. 12. Clinical interfaces of special chart and automatic prescription.

4.2 P2C communication

Before development of the CIPC, prostate cancer patients were tracked by handwriting QOL assessments during cure period but lacks of automatic electronic progress. Because of physical or mental suffering, patients used to complete paper works through conversation with health care people. Meanwhile, doctors took many efforts to explain PROs at clinic time by printing out PCRs for advices. Therefore, the RTCDSS was established by practical requirements on increasing interaction with patients to consolidate relationship as well as reducing official burden of health care people. Following the CIPC procedure mentioned in Fig 3, moreover, all personal data were encrypted as being written into the database to avoid being falsified and stolen. Hence patients have enough confidence under risk avoidance to comply with clinicians' guidance. In the practice, patients read the introduction and login with personal ID to start the QOL assessment. As shown in Fig 13, there's only one question per browser page and the patient can adjust suitable font size on the touched screen in addition to consider the voice control button for assistance. On the other hand, the clinician is able to compare patient's record with others who meet similar markers and evaluate assessment results by figures or charts for advanced consultation.

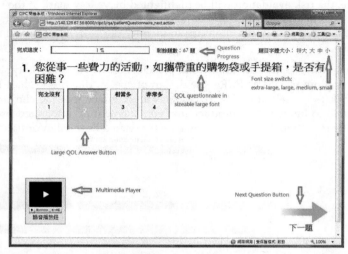

Fig. 13. Screenshot of QOL questionnaire page of CIPC system for prostate cancer patients.

i.   *Cross comparison* – the example chart shown in Fig 14 supports the clinician and patient to take an overview for discussing the variation of QOL compared with the mean value of other patients in similar conditions. It enhanced the patient with confidence to follow doctor's comments for advanced treatment. In the pilot study, patients reflected motivation with more interaction to clinicians as recognizing QOL history with clinical markers.

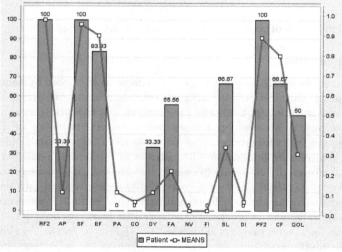

Fig. 14. Cross comparison after assessment (Lin et al., 2010).

ii. *Overall evaluation* – Fig 8 displays the change of QOL, which became better after some particular time because of the successful prostate surgery. Referring the PSA history compared with selected QOL domains, patient's PSA was improved after accepting surgery operation in early 2007. However, a suspected point was observed in the period around July in 2007 under stable PSA baseline, the patient felt uncomfortable since the physical function was suddenly getting worse while the diarrhoea symptom became significant. It assisted the clinician recognizing whether the problem was caused by the prostate disease.

iii. *Real time informetrix categories for patients* – The best practice of the developed system should be applied for patients whose disease can be chronically and periodically tracked by specified clinical markers. Therefore the design of real time infometrix for prostate cancer patients displays their PSA values associated with QOL domains to provide categories of physical, role, cognitive, emotional, and social functions in addition to that of fatigue, pain, nausea and vomiting symptoms. Particularly, it reflects urinary, bowel, treatment-related symptoms and male-related sexual functioning. Patients can recognize personal health condition immediately with respect to others through the instant graphical chart in the clinic.

From aspect of participant clinicians, they use the system mainly for functional assessment as well as for highlighting patients' most bothersome symptoms. The most common benefits would include enhancing communication with patients, identifying under-reported symptoms for clinicians and increasing efficiency in clinics. To assess the advantage of the developed system for users, some interesting problems are observed and discussed below.

i.   *Online informatics for clinicians* – The greatest advantage conferred by this system is its ability to assist in the treatment of chronic diseases that can be periodically tracked using the specific clinical variables as shown in Fig 9. The online informatics displays PSA-related data to provide categories of diagnostic information. Clinicians can identify patients' health conditions directly with respect to treatments through the instant diagrams. The participants reported that the RTCDSS saved hours, even several days, of analysis for them by providing instant computation of the relevant parameters.

ii. *Improvement in clinician-patients relationships* – Several studies in chronic diseases suggested that feedback of health status data may facilitate communication between patients and clinicians to enhance patients' care (Kazis et al., 1990; Wagner et al., 1997). Accordingly, incorporating QOL assessments in routine clinical oncology practice can heighten physicians' awareness of their patients' (Detmar et al., 2002). In the CIPC, clinicians predicted potential disease risk as shown in Fig 10. Thus, the clinician could refer to the interactive guideline in Fig 11 while offering the suggestions, ordering the proper treatment, and tracking the follow-up conditions. Correspondingly, the system assists clinicians to discover reliable QOL information of patients since they would like to confess more factual illness status. The auto-data transportation procedure minimizes manual mistakes to ensure data quality and confirm the RTCDSS has capacity to improve clinician-patient relationships.

iii. *Enhancement in P2C communication* – Both of online infometrics and interactive guideline in routine clinical practice can enhance clinicians' awareness of their patients'. Herein, clinicians use the developed system to discover reliable predictive information for prostate cancer patients through real time statistics and computation. Therefore, manual mistakes can be eliminated by the automatic transportation procedure to ensure data quality. It confirms that the framework of the real time CIPC system is possible and feasible to improve communication between patients and clinicians.

4.3 Advantage and difficulty

The biggest benefits of CIPC system would likely enhance clinical care for patients, support optimal treatment options for clinicians, and increase efficiency in clinics. The advantages of the developed system can be summarized: (a) ensuring quality of clinical care, (b) providing the clinicians real-time online clinical informatics, (c) enhancing P2C communication, and (d) improving clinician-patients relationships. Behind the successes above, however, the past studies also experienced difficulties as practicing the new system restricted by management policies and a flexible strategy is considered to satisfy the actual condition. The hospital management and security policy limited the CIPC system only work partially for proposed clinic beyond the hospital network. As adapting the system to the legacy HIS, noises of diverse systems are always counted for integration. The structural reformation on original HIS should be avoidant but through gradual data immigration under administration rules.

Herein, the CIPC system was installed in the server at the urology clinics in which an individual patient used to make appointment on a specific day of week. In compliance with hospital management for safety policy, the power of clinic room was turned off after clinics and the CIPC server must be shutdown. To avoid conflicting with the HIS but ensure data transformation can synchronize between inconsistent systems, a process scheduling module was employed for data importation between the HIS and CIPC system. The module was embedded in both systems to retrieve required data from the backup log of CIPC system at a specified time point and transform data into the HIS database. As a result, clinicians could obtain the last patient outcomes if their data were imported into the HIS just before clinic time. Fig 15 illustrates three data-update jobs in a cycle as considering two scheduling points

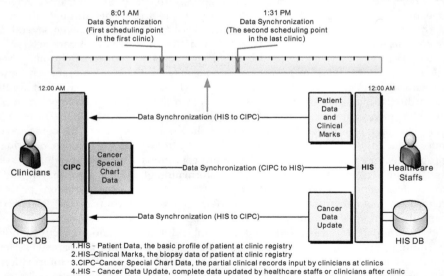

Fig. 15. Processes scheduling of data transformation for heterogeneous system integration.

before and after the clinics. At the first point in the first clinic, the required data are replicated into the backup log. In the cycle, clinicians activate the start button to load PCRs and clinical markers from the log into CIPC database; and then, the new outcomes will be input during clinic time. After the clinic, clinicians can update complete remarks of PCR to CIPC database and all data will be restored to the backup log concurrently. At the second point in the last clinic, the log will be retrieved in schedule and be transformed into the HIS. Once the CIPC server is activated, the scheduling will be automatically started. In the study, the process scheduling was executed twice per week by urological clinics. The "quasi real time" strategy above can help solving the difficulty while implementing a new development into the legacy system under management restriction.

4.4 Practice discussions

The system confers the following benefits: (1) clinicians can explain health conditions clearly to patients by visualized clinical variables and pretreatment parameters; (2) patients are more easily convinced by evidence-based diagrams before accepting the risk evaluation of treatments and the treatment quality can be confirmed; (3) the design presents real-time disease and risk evaluation while the interactive guidelines with treatment suggestions offer the clinician efficient online tools for instant decision making; (4) the proposed framework is constructed upon the Web-based MVC architecture that consists of reusable models, making it flexible and adaptable with many hospital information systems. In the pilot study, more than 90% of users approved the innovative design. Clinicians learned more reliable information regarding patient's private QOL. The efficient diagnosis and communication certainly encourages the advanced study. With RTCDSS for predicting treatment assistance, diverse functionalities can be expectant for advance clinical decision, context-specific access, automatic risk assessment, personal digital assistant screens, as well as practitioner performance and cost-effectiveness on patient outcomes (Aaronson et al., 1993). In the future, the real-time decision support functions can be expanded flexibly by involving other diagnostic variables and modern technologies like RNA and DNA studies. It can also incorporate with advanced prediction models such as nomograms, which may help patients and their treating physicians make informed decisions based on the probability of a pathologic stage, the patient's risk tolerance, and the values they place on the various potential outcomes (Stephenson et al., 2005). The system will aid the rational selection of patients to undergo definitive therapy.

5. Conclusion remarks

This study reveals clinical and infometrics progress with information technology to establish fundamentals of the RTCDSS. Methodologies include MVC architecture, Web services, online analytical process, clinical data warehouse, object relation mapping, and AJAX while the practical CIPC system is implemented for approval. The infrastructure integrates five layers to establish expandable models with flexibility for providing accessible functions in clinic applications of prostate cancer. Heterogeneous database systems distributed in hospital, clinic and campus networks were integrated for an expert bank with remote data backup and disaster recovery. A patient- and clinician-oriented interface is considered as a major subject to assist P2C communication. In advance, the patient outcome is available to offer instant statistical charts for decision making as well as improved communication and relationship between clinicians and patients. Furthermore, the RTCDSS enables interactive guideline for knowledge feedback, facilitate decision-making, and to improve quality of care.

6. Acknowledgment

The author sincerely appreciates Professors Hsi-Chin Wu, Chih-Hung Chang, Tsai-Chung Li, Wen-Miin Liang, and Jong-Yi Wang for their encouragements and consultants. The author also thanks IT-engineer Yu-Yuan Chou and Statistician Yi-Chun Yeh as well as Biostatistics Center of China Medical University for their help in statistical analysis and informatics support. This study was granted by National Science Council and China Medical University with projects no. NSC100-2625-M-039-001, CMU96-153, CMU96-228, and CMU97-321.

7. References

Aaronson, N.K., et al. (1993). The European Organization for Research and Treatment of Cancer QLQ-C30: A quality-of-Life Instrument for use in International clinical trials in oncology, *J. Nat'l Cancer Institute*, 85:365-376.

Bauger, C. & King, G. (2005) "Hibernate in Action," in *Manning Publications*, Shelter Island, New York.

Bazinet, M., et al. (1994). Prospective evaluation of prostate-specific antigen density and systematic biopsies for early detection of prostatic carcinoma, Urology, 43:44-51.

Carter, H.B., et al. (1992). Longitudinal evaluation of prostate-specific antigen levels in men with and without prostate disease, *JAMA*, 267:2215-2220.

Carter, H.B., Allae, M.E., Partin, A.W. (2007). Diagnosis and Staging of Prostate Cancer, in Sec.XVI, Ch.94, *Campbell-Walsh Urology*. Vol.3. 9th ed. Edited by Wein AJ. Philadelphia: W.B. Saunders.

Chang, C., et al. (2007). A System for Interactive Assessment and Management in Palliative Care, *J. Pain and Symptom Management*, 33:745-755.

Chang, C. (2008). Novel Pain Assessment and Intervention Network (NoPAIN) and Clinical Infometrics. *J. Pain*, 8:S72-S72.

Chaudhuri, S. & Dayal, U. (1997). An Overview of Data Warehousing and OLAP Technology, *ACM SIGMOD Record*, 26(1):65-74.

D'Amico, A.V., et al. (2001). Predicting prostate specific antigen outcome preoperatively in the prostate specific antigen era, *J. Urol.*, 166:2185-2188.

D'Amico, A.V., Renshaw, A.A., Sussman, B., Chen, M.H. (2005). Pretreatment PSA velocity and risk of death from prostate cancer following external beam radiation therapy, *JAMA*, 294:440-447.

Dorfman, C.S., et al. (2010). The development of a web- and a print-based decision aid for prostate cancer screening, *BMC Med. Inform. Decis. Mak.*, 10:12, URL: www.biomedcentral.com/1472-6947/10/12.

Detmar, S.B., Muller, M.J., Schornagel, J.H., Wever, L.D.V., Aaronson, N.K. (2002). Health-related quality-of-life assessments and patient-physician communication: a randomized controlled trial, *JAMA*, 288(23):3027-3034.

Ercole, C.J., et al. (1987). Prostatic specific antigen and prostatic acid phosphatase in the monitoring and staging of patients with prostatic cancer, *J. Urology*, 138:1181-1184.

Fowler, J.E., et al. (1994). Prostate specific antigen progression rates after radical prostatectomy or radiation therapy for localized prostate cancer, *Surg.*, 116:302-306.

Freifeld, C.C., Mandl, K.D., Reis, B.Y., Brownstein, J.S. (2008). HealthMap: global Infectious Disease Monitoring through Automated Classification and Visualization of internet media reports, *J. Am. Med. Info. Assoc.*, 15(2):150-157.

Fung, C.F., Lim, Y.W., Mattke, S., Damberg, C., Shekelle, P.G. (2008). Systematic Review: The Evidence That Publishing Patient Care Performance Data Improves Quality of Care. *Annals of Internal Medicine*, 148(2):111-123.

Gamma, E., Helm, R., Johnson, R., Vlissides, J. (1994). *Design Patterns: Elements of Reusable Object-Oriented Software*, Addison-Wesley.

Gann, P.H., Hennekens, C.H., Stampfer, M.J. (1995). A prospective evaluation of plasma prostate-specific antigen for detection of prostatic cancer, *JAMA*, 273:289-294.

Gleason, D. (1966). Classification of prostatic carcinoma, *Cancer Chemother Rep.*, 50(3):125-128.

Gottschalk, K., Graham, S., Kreger, H., Snell, J. (2002). Introduction to Web Services Architecture, *IBM Systems Journal*, 41(2):170-177.

Holmes-Rovner, M., et al. (2005). Evidence-based patient choice: a prostate cancer decision aid in plain language, *BMC Med. Inform. Decis. Mak.*, 5:16, URL: www.biomedcentral.com/1472-6947/5/16/.

Hsu, J., et al. (2005). Health information technology and physician-patient interactions: impact of computers on communication during outpatient primary care visits, *J. Am. Med. Info. Assoc.*, 12(4):474-480.

Hunt, D.L., Haynes, R.B., Hanna, S.E., Smith, K. (1998). Effects of Computer-Based Clinical Decision Support Systems on Physician Performance and Patient Outcomes, *JAMA*, 280:1339-1346.

Inmon, B. & Kelley, C. (1994). The Twelve Rules of Data Warehouse for a Client/Server World," *Data Management Review*, 4(5):6-16.

Johnston, M.E., Langton, K.B., Haynes, R.B., Mathieu, A. (1994). Effects of Computer-based Clinical Decision Support Systems on Clinician Performance and Patient Outcome: A Critical Appraisal of Research. *J. Internal Medicine*, 120:135-142.

Kaplan, E.L. & Meier, P. (1958). Nonparametric estimation from incomplete observations, *J. Am. Stat. Assoc.*, 53:457-481.

Kazis, L.E., Callahan, L.F., Meenan, R.F., Pincus, T. (1990). Health status reports in the care of patients with rheumatoid arthritis," *J. Clinic Epidemiology*, 43(11):1243-1253.

Kleer, E. & Oesterling, J.E. (1993). PSA and staging of localized prostate cancer, *J. Urol. Clin. North Am.*, 20:695-704.

Krasner, G.E. & Pope, S.T. (1988). A cookbook for using the model-view-controller user interface paradigm in Smalltalk-80, *J. Object-Oriented Programming*, 1(3):26-49.

Liem, E.B., Obeid, J.S., Shareck, E.P., Sato, L., Greenes, R.A. (1995). Representation of clinical practice guidelines through an interactive world-wide-web interface, *Proc. Annu. Symp. Comput. Appl. Med. Care*, 223-227.

Lin, H.-C., et al. (2010). A Real Time Online Assessment System with Modelized Architecture on Clinical Infometrics for Patient Reported Outcomes of Prostate Cancer. *Computer Methods and Programs in Biomedicine*, in press, doi:10.1016/j.cmpb.2010.10.003.

Lin, H.-C., et al. (2011). Development of a Real-Time Clinical Decision Support System upon the Web MVC-based Architecture for Prostate Cancer Treatment, *BMC Med. Inform. Decis. Mak.*, 11:16, URL: www.biomedcentral.com/1472-6947/11/16.

Maviglia, S.M., Zielstorff, R.D., Paterno, M., Teich, J.M., Bates, D.W., Kuperman, G.J. (2003). Automating complex guidelines for chronic disease: lessons learned, *J. Am. Med. Info. Assoc.*, 10:154-165.

Moulding, N.T., Silagy, C.A., Weller, D.P. (1999). A framework for effective management of change in clinical practice: dissemination and implementation of clinical practice guidelines, *Quality in Health Care*, 8:177-183.

Rob, P. & Cornel, C. (2004). "Database Systems: Design, Implementation and Management, Chapter 12, *Tomson Course Technology*, 6th ed.

Partin, A.W., et al. (1993). The use of prostate specific antigen, clinical stage and Gleason score to predict pathological stage in men with localized prostate cancer, *J. Urol.*, 150:110-114.

Partin, A.W., et al. (1997). Combination of prostate-specific antigen, clinical stage, and Gleason score to predict pathological stage of localized prostate cancer. A multi-institutional update, *JAMA*, 277:1445-1451.

Partin, A.W., et al. (2001). Contemporary update of prostate cancer staging nomograms (Partin tables) for the new millennium, *J. Urology*, 58:843-848.

Pound, C.R., et al. (1999). Natural history of progression after PSA elevation following radical prostatectomy, *JAMA*, 281:1591-1597.

Sanders, G., Nease, R.F.Jr., Owens, D.K. (2001). Publishing web-based guidelines using interactive decision models, *J. Eval. Clin. Pract.*, 7(2):175-189.

Sensabaugh, G. F. (1978). Isolation and characterization of a semen-specific protein from human seminal plasma: a potential new marker for semen identification, *J. Forensic Sci.*, 23:106-115.

Shiffman, R.N., et al. (2000). GEM: a proposal for a more comprehensive guideline document model using XML, *J. Am. Med. Info. Assoc.*, 7:488-498.

Smith, K. (2006). Simplifying Ajax-style Web development, Computer, 39(5):98-101.

Stephenson, A.J., et al. (2005). Postoperative Nomogram Predicting the 10-Year Probability of Prostate Cancer Recurrence After Radical Prostatectomy, *J. Clinical Oncology*, 23(28):7005-7012.

Uzzo, R.G., et al. (1995). The influence of prostate size on cancer detection, *J. Urol.* 46:831-836.

Walter, L.C. & Covinsky, K.E. (2001). Cancer Screening in Elderly Patients - A Framework for Individualized Decision Making, *JAMA*, 285:2750-2756.

Wang, M.C., et al. (1981). Prostate antigen: A new potential marker for prostatic cancer, *The Prostate*, 2(1):89-96.

Wagner, A.K., et al. (1997). Patient-based health status measurement in clinical practice: a study of its impact on epilepsy patients' care, *Quality of Life Research*, 6(4):329-341.

Zielstorff, R.D. (1998). Online practice guidelines issues, obstacles, and future prospects, *J. Am. Med. Info. Assoc.*, 5:227-236.

6

Wireless Monitoring of Patient's Vital Signs

Anna G. C. D. Ribeiro[1], André L. Maitelli[1], Ricardo A. M. Valentim[1],
Cicília Raquel Maia Leite[2] and Ana M. G. Guerreiro[1]
[1]Laboratory of Hospital Automation and Bioengineering,
Federal University of Rio Grande do Norte,
[2]State University of Rio Grande do Norte,
Brazil

1. Introduction

With all the technological advances and current devices available, large and good projects are not only restricted to the invention of new technologies and concepts but also, and mainly, to the merging of existing technologies resulting in new ideas and devices that address problems not yet solved.

Mobile computing and portable devices, for example, are changing the relationships between human and computers, and are introducing a new approach of communication based on context. According to Figueiredo (Figueiredo & Nakamura, 2003) this new approach of communication allows people to interact seamlessly with objects, computers, environments, etc. Such technological advances are a significant departure from the existing computational paradigm in which users need to interact explicitly with the systems in order to achieve the expected results.

This new paradigm, known as Ubiquitous Computing, named by Weiser (Weiser, 1991), has the ability to foster a different computer vision, focusing on people's daily life (and daily tasks). Its current applications and future possibilities can be utilized in an almost invisible way, allowing the user to communicate with technology without even realizing it. Thus, the processes occur for the user, as the services and interfaces are hiding the complexity of the system.

The medical field, in its constant pursuit for finding new methods of healing and improving patients' quality of life, has been, and will continue to be, a major beneficiary of Ubiquitous Computing. Although not a substitute for the direct contact between physician and patient, is increasingly becoming an essential and indispensable factor for physician's decision-making. The current telemedicine systems provide global integration, which enables the sharing of data, images and voice from different sources and applications.

This chapter proposal describes how wireless technologies can be used in medicine, offering many benefits to doctors and patients including new methods of surgery, appointments or monitoring. It presents a review of the current medical situation and how it can be improved using new technologies.

Patient monitoring is indispensible to any hospital. Any Intensive Care Unit (ICU) or hospital beds are surrounded by electrical devices monitoring the patient and these devices are often responsible for saving a patient life. Due to the importance of these devices, there are many studies in how to improve the monitoring and they are focused specially in three questions: What, where and when should it be monitored? The obvious answer would be: everything, everywhere, every time, but in many cases that is not possible.

Studies show that a good way to have an overview of the patient health is through the vital signs (Lima, 2002), and not only patients admitted to the ICU require continuous follow-up of those signs. There are many patients with chronic or debilitating diseases who do not need to remain in the hospital but, nonetheless, need constant monitoring of their vitals to assist in early detection of dangerous situations(Kochar & Woods, 1990) (Mion et. al, 2004). At the same time that more developed countries are thriving with all these technological advancements, third world countries have been struggling with insufficient ICU beds. In Brazil, for example, the number of ICU beds has been increasing at a significantly lower rate than the one recommended by the WHO (World Health Organization). (OMS, 2009) Thus, there has been a significant increase in the number of homecare systems offered around the world. However, while they provide an interesting alternative to communities facing health care challenges, most of those solutions still have important limitations, in particular for patients facing more debilitating conditions, such as Alzheimer, Parkinson, and physical disabilities. Those patients need a new way of care monitoring that can bring increased comfort and security for themselves and their families.

Given this problem, this chapter proposes a wireless monitoring of patient's vital signs, presenting a new telemedicine software using GPRS (General Packet Radio Service) and Bluetooth technologies that adds the idea of ubiquity to the medical area, innovating the relation between doctor and patient through wireless communication and bringing security and confidence to a patient being monitored in homecare.

2. Ubiquitous computing

Ubiquitous computing aims to make human-computer interaction invisible, i.e., integrating computing with personal   actions and behavior. (Sousa, 2002). Ubiquitous computing is roughly the opposite of virtual reality. Where virtual reality puts people inside a computer-generated world, ubiquitous computing forces the computer to live out here in the world with people. Virtual reality is primarily a horse power problem; ubiquitous computing is a very difficult integration of human factors, computer science, engineering, and social sciences.

The last 50 years of computing can be divided into two major trends: the mainframe, with many people sharing a computer, and computers with a personal computer for each user (Fig 1) . Since 1984 the number of people using PCs is greater than the number of people sharing computers. The next era would be of Ubiquitous Computing (Ubicomp also called), with many computers, embedded in walls, furniture, clothes and cars, sharing each one of us.

Ubiquitous computing (Fig 2) is defined as the junction of two other concepts that are: Mobile Computing, where a computing device and its services can be relocated while they are connected in a network or the Internet. The other is the Pervasive Computing, in which computing devices are distributed in the environment in a seamlessly way (Weiser, 1996).

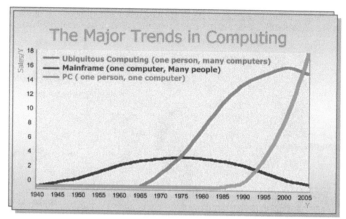

Fig. 1. Trends in computing.

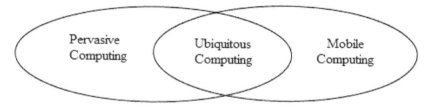

Fig. 2. Ubiquitous computing.

Pervasive computing: This concept states that media will be distributed in the working environment for users in a noticeable or perceptible way (Hess,2002). Through this concept, it is assumed that the computer would be distributed in the environment, and it would be only one machine on the table. Equipped with sensors, the computer would be able to detect and extract data and environmental variations, automatically generating computer models controlling, configuring and tuning applications as the needs of users and other devices. As this interaction, each member of the set would be able to detect the mutual presence of both users of other devices, and automatically interact among them building a intelligent framework for better usability (Fig 3).

Mobile computing: It is the ability of a computing device and the services associated with it are mobile, allowing it to be loaded or transported staying connected to the network or the Internet.

It is verified this concept today in the use of wireless networks, Internet access via mobile devices or even via the phone itself. We can also check the growth of Bluetooth applications through headphones, wireless photo printers or wireless mice.

Thus, as shown in Fig 2, ubiquitous computing benefits from the technological advances of both branches of research. Therefore, ubiquity is the integration between mobility and

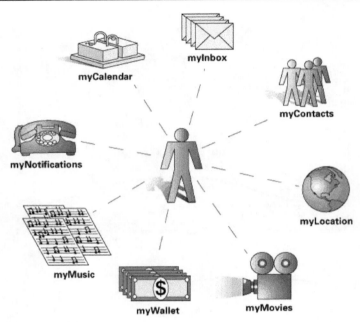

Fig. 3. Pervasive computing.

presence systems with distributed, largely invisible, intelligent and highly integrated computers and their applications for the benefit of users. This junction arise the concepts of:

- Disaggregated Computing: dynamic reconfiguration of the interface devices. Example: the ability to make your presentation move to any screen in the room. The "computer" is a diverse group of connected devices, which are actually attached to different computers on the network.
- Position Sensitive Computing: interaction with computers changes as people move. Example: Auto tour guide in a museum, automatically move your desktop to the closest display, as you walk around the room.
- Augmented Reality: Combine Wearable computers with information from position sensors, the user's relevant information can be superimposed in real vision of the world. This view can be displayed over helmets coupled with displays or even through special glasses, allowing the user to have access to an Augmented Reality. Unlike Virtual Reality (VR), where only the information generated by computer is displayed, Augmented Reality is a combination of VR with the actual image. For practical purposes this technology could be employed, for example, military sights on long-range weapons or civilly in identification, displaying or enhancing the user information out of the reach of his normal vision.
- Sensitive Object Interfaces: physical objects associated to some information. Example: to associate an object to the web page of your manufacturer. Perhaps the technology closer to reality, been used in some supermarkets in the U.S. and Europe and some production lines through RFID systems (Radio Frequency Identification).

"The deepest and most enduring technologies are those that disappear. They dissipate in the things of everyday life until they become indistinguishable."(Weiser, 1991)

Mark Weiser (Weiser, 1996) proposal is becoming a reality, through technologies such as PDAs, smart-phones, and the consolidation of wireless networking standards such as Bluetooth (Bluetooth.org 2004) and IEEE 802.11 (IEEE 2005). With ubiquitous computing, the relationship between users and computing devices changes compared to personal computers, what it was one to one, happens to be one to many (one user to multiple devices).

In addition to mobility, ubiquitous systems support interoperability, scalability, among other things to ensure that users have access when they want (Fig 4). According to Saha and Mukherjee (Saja & Mukherjee 2003), advances in technology necessary to build a ubiquitous computing environment are: devices, interconnection network, middleware, and applications.

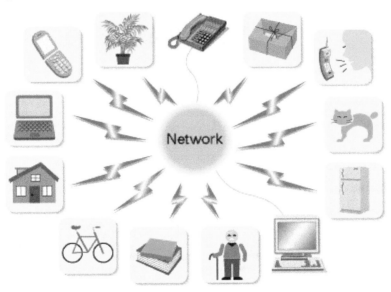

Fig. 4. Ubiquitous Computing , access everywhere.

2.1 Ubiquitous medicine

The development of technologies for health care are becoming a recurring term in the research field, whether the field of Engineering, Exact Sciences, Health or Human Sciences. This aspect characterizes the development of technology in health as a transversal element, or even transdisciplinary, for whose purpose is to study innovation in health usually permeate the border areas of knowledge, a factor that almost require interdisciplinary or transdisciplinary (Guimarães, 2004).

Health care seems to be an ideal application field for ubiquitous computing. Where else is the paradigm of "getting the right information at the right time at the right place of greater importance than in health care? Scenarios for application of ubiquitous computing are home care and monitoring, assistance for health professionals, and the self organization of health care institutions. Wearable systems and especially new man-machine interfaces are key technologies of ubiquitous computing in health care . Another key technology, namely RFID chips (Radio Frequency Identification) (Stanford, 2003), useful for realizing context awareness of ubiquitous computing solutions is already available and in use in several domains. These miniaturized chips allow the wireless transfer of data within a limited area around a special RFID reader and can be used to identify nearby people and objects.

Ubiquitous medical environments are those in which technological advances such as mobile devices and wireless networks bring new opportunities for access and interaction of its users, such as access of patient information. This information makes up the so-called Electronic Patient Record (EPR), allowing data about tests, facts and situations concerning the health of a patient to be accessed through multiple devices and heterogeneous networks. Ubiquitous in medicine can be made to EPRs access to consolidated information on patients from anywhere in the network, allowing also cooperation between professionals regardless the time and space. In particular, medical ubiquitous environments must support the mobility of its employees, given that mobility is inherent in the medical profession. In addition to this nomadic nature of the doctor, it is important to consider that the medical activity is highly fragmented, i.e., shall be subject to interruptions during execution, as doctors spend little time at each location or activity. Thus, mechanisms that facilitate the professional's activities tend to improve their productivity. The importance of ubiquitous computing occurs not only when the main actor is the doctor, it can also be applied in the "world" of the patient, optimizing, for example, their monitoring system. Therefore the proposal shown in this chapter is not only a EPR system modernized but also the implementation of a unique module for tracking and monitoring patients.

2.2 Patient monitoring

Patient monitoring systems comprise sensors, data communication, storage, processing, and presentation of medical data. These functions are performed both near the patient, in local surgery, or remotely at a health care infrastructure, e.g., a medical centre or a hospital. Patient monitoring systems can be used in a variety of health care scenarios ranging from paramedic, diagnostic, surgical, post-operative, and home surveillance situations. The systems must meet a high demand of flexibility since data may be produced outside a health care enterprise (Maghsudi et. Al, 199) ((Raffloer & Wiggens, 1997). This requires specific measures in order to fulfill security, availability, privacy, and Quality of Service (QoS) demands. The properties are: a) mobility; b) outside hospital infrastructure; c) biomedical sensor networks in use; d) wireless channel.

2.2.1 Home care monitoring

Among the factors that drive the advancement of home care are: advanced treatments for many diseases and scientific technology resulting in rising costs of hospital care, increased the incidence of chronic degenerative and mental diseases determining the need for continued assistance; risks of cross infection, highly competitive world market; early hospital discharge with short periods of hospital stay.

There are three forms of service at home. The first is to domiciliary hospitalization, i.e., a patient transferred from hospital to home. In this type of assistance, it requires continuous monitoring, and sometimes, uninterrupted, 24, 12, 8 or 6 hours of nursing care. It is essential the continued support with a call center solution for emergencies, 24 hours, with doctors and nurses available to guide and fulfill the needs of the patient (e.g., patient dependent on mechanical ventilation, intravenous therapy and total dependence on nursing care).

The second type assists patients not totally dependent, who constitute the large majority. These patients require relatively complex procedures, with up to 3 hours of care provided at his home by a professional team. It is generally directed to patients unable to attend to medical treatment because they are bedridden and dependent on oxygen therapy, and other pathologies. Many of them only require specific care such as daily dressings, intramuscularly or intravenously medication. For these services the frequency of home visits is determined by the professional team.

The third method is the monitoring of patients with chronic diseases such as diabetes mellitus, hypertension, among others, through the implementation of health education, beyond the control and guidance. Thus it avoids re-hospitalizations or aggravations of health status, and provides safety and comfort for patients and their families.

The increase in life expectancy in recent years has led to the world an increasingly aging population. The problem is not aging, but aging with no quality of life. The overcrowding of health services is consequential, as well as the social security problems. The home care comes to help treat chronic and stable patients, and one of the goals is to take the patient to the hospital and treat him at home. It is less expensive for the public service and less cumbersome for the patient, who could spend months or years in a hospital since his illness is chronic and / or degenerative. The home care reduces exposure to risk of hospital infections, reduces costs and encourages the rotation of beds in hospitals, especially cases of chronic-degenerative or extensive postoperative. In addition, in most cases the availability of beds in hospitals is small. The home care also offers the possibility of a treatment with appropriate technology, highly trained professionals and family environment. (Krupinski et. al. ,2002)

3. Wireless communication systems

One of the biggest challenges of patient monitoring outside the hospital is their mobility, since the incumbent technology requires them to be connected to machines within a room. Nowadays, this issue can be addressed with the use of cell phones.

According to the Brazilian Telecommunication Agency (Anatel, 2011), Brazil has 175.6 million mobile phones and the teledensity (number of phone lines per 100 inhabitants) has reached 91.33 in February 2010. Mobile phones are used not only to make and receive calls, but also to send and receive data, having become an option for Internet access Furthermore, with the advent of wireless technologies, such as Bluetooth, mobile devices can communicate with other devices and computers. The trend is that the mobile phone will replace several technologies currently on the market (Fig 5).

That makes the cell phone an excellent option for patient monitoring: it allows for the desired patient mobility with full access to the internet (central sever). For the full mobility, the monitor and sensors must also be mobile (e.g. wearable for continuous monitoring).

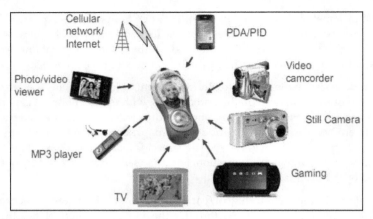

Fig. 5. Technologies convergence.

3.1 GPRS (General Packet Radio Service)

The GPRS (General Packet Radio) is a technology that increases data transfer rates on existing GSM networks. This allows the transport of packet data (packet switching). Thus, the GPRS provides a data transfer rate much higher than previous technologies, which used circuit switching, which were around 12Kbps. Since the GPRS, in ideal situations, exceed the mark of 170kbps. However in practice this rate is around 40 kbps (Comtech M2M, 2011).

Unlike circuit switching technology, the GPRS service is "always on", i.e. it is a mode in which resources are only assigned to a user when necessary to send or receive data. This enables operators to provide access to the GPRS mobile internet at high speed and at reasonable cost, because the charge is the amount of data packets transmitted and not for connect time on the network. Because it uses packet switching, GPRS phones do not require dedicated circuits allocated to itself. Dynamically a physical channel is established, it remains while data is being transmitted and can be assigned to another user so that the transmission is completed, making more efficient use of network. The Fig 6 shows that we can transmit the data to the internet through a mobile phone by using a GPRS.

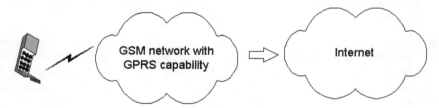

Fig. 6. Transmitting data to the internet through GPRS capability.

3.2 Bluetooth

Bluetooth is a global standard for wireless communication and low power consumption that allows data transmission between compatible devices with the technology. For this, a data combination of hardware and software is used to allow this communication to occur between the most different types of devices. Data transmission is done through radio frequency, allowing a device to detect the other regardless of their positions, since they remain within the limit of proximity. To be able to meet all kinds of devices, Bluetooth's maximum range was divided into three classes (Bluetooth, 2011):

Class 1: maximum power of 100 mW, range up to 100 meters;
Class 2: maximum power of 2.5 mW, range up to 10 meters;
Class 3: maximum power of 1 mW, range up to 1 meter.

This means that a device with Bluetooth class 3 will only be able to communicate with another if the distance between them is less than 1 meter, for example. In this case, the distance may seem useless, but it is enough to connect a headset to a mobile phone hanging on the waist of one person. It is worth noting, however, that different classes of devices can communicate without any problem, by simply respecting the limit of the one that has a smaller range. The speed of data transmission in Bluetooth is low: up to version 1.2, the rate can reach up to 1 Mbps. In version 2.0, this value increased to up to 3 Mbps. Although these rates are short, are sufficient for a data successful connection between most of the devices. However, the search for higher speeds is constant, as evidenced by the arrival of version 3.0, capable of rates up to 24 Mbps (Diane,2002).

Bluetooth is a technology designed to work around the world, which is why it was necessary to adopt one open radio frequency, which is standard anywhere in the world. The ISM band (Industrial, Scientific, Medical), that operates at a frequency of 2.45 GHz, it is the closest of this necessity and is used in several countries, with variations ranging from 2.4 to 2.5 GHz. As a device communicating via Bluetooth can both receive and transmit data (full-duplex mode), the transmission switches between transmit and receive slots, a scheme known as FH / TDD (Frequency Hopping / Time-Division Duplex). These channels are divided into slots of 625 ms periods (microseconds). Each frequency should be filled by a slot, so in one second, has 1,600 jumps.

The goal of Bluetooth is to allow intercommunication of nearby devices using the lowest possible power consumption (especially because many of these devices are powered by batteries) and a low implementation cost.

3.3 J2ME (Java Micro Edition)

Java Micro Edition is a set of APIs (Application Programming Interface) for developing Java application for mobile phones, J2ME is supported at least by most brands of mobile phones such as Motorola, Nokia, Panasonic and others.

The main components of the Java 2 Platform, Micro Edition (J2ME platform) is the CDC (Connected Device Configurations, connected devices), the CLDC (Connected Limited Device Configurations, for devices with limited connection), the MIDP (Mobile Information Device Profiles Profiles of information from mobile devices), plus many other tools and technologies that bring solutions to consumer markets in Java and embedded devices. There are three types of virtual machine for Java (Fig 7):

• JVM (for desktop computers);

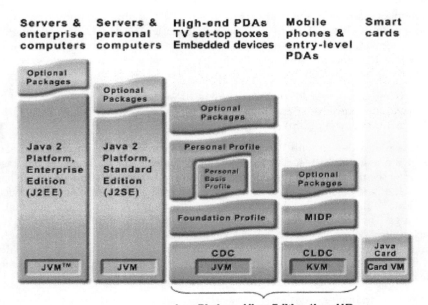

Fig. 7. Java hierarchy. (Java, 2011)

- KVM (for mobile phones and PDA's);
- and JavaCard VM (for Smartcards).

The program made in Java (J2ME) is called a MIDlet. MIDlet is a Java application for mobile devices, more specifically the J2ME virtual machine. In general applications are to run on phones, such as games and others. MIDlets will (should) run on any device that implements J2ME MIDP. Like all Java programs, MIDlets are fully portable and made to run on any platform. To write a MIDlet, you can get the Sun's Wireless Toolkit Java site, which is available for multiple platforms and is free.

A MIDlet has the following requirements to run on a mobile phone:

- The main class must be subclass of javax.microedition.midlet.MIDlet;
- A MIDlet must be packaged in a arquivo.jar (eg using the jar-tool)
- The. Jar file needs to be pre-checked.

4. Angel care mobile system

This section presents a software development that meets the needs mentioned above and aims to improve physician and patient lives through better homecare and web monitoring.

4.1 System architecture

The *AngelCare* solution (Ribeiro et. al. , 2010) was developed in Java ME (Java Micro Edition) for mobile devices and it is responsible for monitoring biomedical signals of a patient in homecare and for sending patient information to a web server on a regular basis. The web server plays the role of a supervisor, storing patient information for online access and sending alerts about the patient's status whenever appropriate.

The system architecture is shown in Fig 8 which describes two scenarios: the patient at home (Communication via Bluetooth) and patient in the hospital (communication via Ethernet).

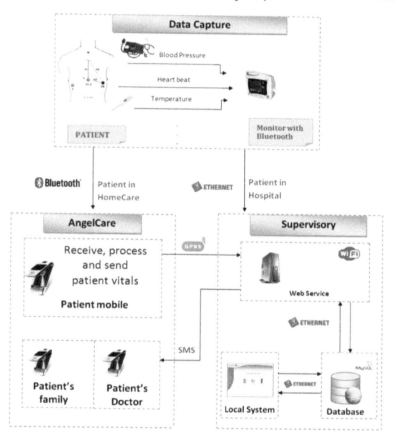

Fig. 8. System Architecture.

If the patient is in hospital, the communication between devices takes place via the local network through the IEEE 802.3 for wired LAN or IEEE 802.11 for wireless communications (Wi-Fi). If the patient is out of the hospital, the monitoring is done by the AngelCare system using Bluetooth and GPRS (General Packet Radio Service).

The architecture illustrated in Fig 8 shows the following components:

- Data Capture: signal transmission with Bluetooth output and Ethernet (IEEE 802.3), responsible for signals capture and transmission;
- AngelCare system with cell phones using Bluetooth and GPRS;

- The supervisory system including the central server that manages all hospital systems, and the system of medical records, on local system, to store information and query the database.

4.2 System modules

The system has three main modules: (i) signal processing and transmission; (ii) alert dispatch; and (iii) database management, as shown in Fig 9.

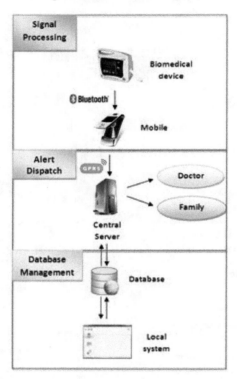

Fig. 9. System modules.

The first module, **signal processing,** the biomedical device connected to the patient communicates with his/her cell phone via Bluetooth technology and sends the data (vital signs) to the phone. It's important to note that each signal has its transmission period because some signals as heart rate needs to be monitored more frequently than body temperature, for example, as the temperature takes more time to change than the heart beat. So, if the device is monitoring signals with different time samples there are 2 solutions, either send them separately or send them together repeating the measure for those that has bigger sample time. In this case, we are sending all together with 3 minutes interval.

When the patient's vital signs reach the cell phone, they are evaluated and compared with the patient's baseline, which had been previously registered in the system, as each patient has different pattern of measurement, so it is necessary to have a previously knowledge about the patient healthy and data.

The purpose of this comparison is to detect potential abnormalities, such as arrhythmia, high/low blood pressure, and abnormal oxygen saturation as shown in Fig 11. If a problem is detected, the data is sent immediately to the web server (supervisor) via GPRS. If there is no abnormality in the patient's signs, the data is packaged in the cellular buffer and sent to the server every six hours, allowing all biomedical signals to be stored for future reference. Once the abnormality is founded not only the actual data is sent, but also, the data saved on the buffer until the present moment (Fig 10).

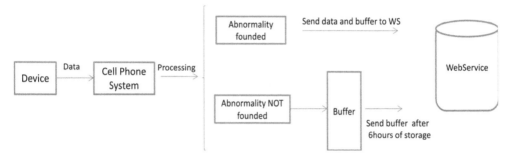

Fig. 10. Event diagram of sending data from the mobile to the web service.

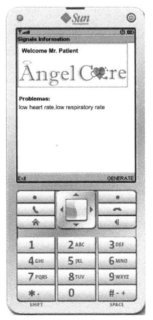

Fig. 11. System showing the patient's abnormalities.

It is important to note that one of the critical enablers of AngelCare's success is the use of GPRS technology, since it allows for sending and receiving information through a mobile telephone network, Global System for Mobile Communications (GSM), with great availability and extended coverage.

The second module, alert dispatch, is triggered whenever the data sent by AngelCare (cell phone) reaches the web server. The monitoring central or health insurance central receives a warning coming from the patient's mobile phone, containing data with the last vitals captured. At that time, the operator should decide on the most appropriated response, such as sending an ambulance to the patient's house or calling the patient's doctor. The server also sends alerts via SMS (Short Message Service) to the patient's family and doctor whenever necessary as the Fig 12 shows.

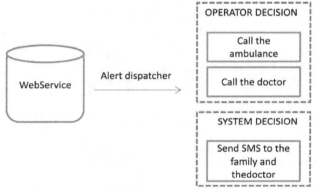

Fig. 12. Alert dispatcher schema.

The third module, database management, deals with storing and retrieving the patient's medical history, including appointments, exams, visits to the emergency room, hospitalizations, etc. All that information is stored in the database and can be accessed through an online platform provided by the system. Fig 13 shows one screen of the online system.

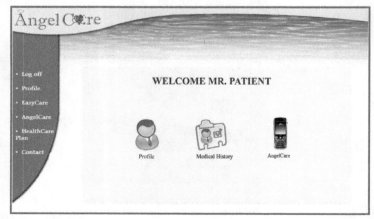

Fig. 13. Online system. Profile Screen.

With the online system the doctor and the patient can access medical history from previous appointments and exams and medical history from the AngelCare monitoring system in case the patient has this feature. The mainly benefit is to access these information anytime and anywhere.

5. Tests and results

This section shows some tests performed with the system and its results. It is focused on the constraints that must be obeyed when it comes to patient monitoring such as time consuming.

There are several reasons to use the mobile phone to process and send the biomedical data. First, it is necessary that the system is self-sufficient and independent from communications network that can fail. A mobile phone is a technology that allows the call center to be constantly updated on the status of the patient, anytime, anywhere.

Secondly, the cellular network also avoids problems related to hospital data traffic, since transmission infrastructure is estimated according to what is being requested .This is a critical point because it is necessary to ensure that the data flow time do not exceed the restrictions imposed by the processes of patients monitoring.

In this context, to prove the viability of the system, some tests analyzing the timing/duration of data transmission were performed.

The data packet generated by the patient's vital signs has 30 bytes. To be on the safe side, all tests were performed with 64 bytes packets, more than double the actual. The timing tests were divided in three steps:

- Data transmission time via Bluetooth from the monitor to the cellular;
- Processing time on the cell phone (used to compare the patient's actual vital signs and its baseline) and;
- Data transmission time from the cellular to the server via GPRS.

Thus, it was possible to analyze the system performance, checking the time spent in each stage the process. To carry out the analysis, 100 tests were performed for each step.

5.1 Bluetooth transmission time

In order to obtain an estimative of the total time of transmission occurred during the transmission of the packet from the biomedical devices to the mobile phone via Bluetooth, it was used RTT (Round Trip Time), which corresponds to the time spent in a round-trip message travels through the network. Thus, through the equation 1 was possible to perform this calculation.

$$T_G = \frac{RTT}{2} \tag{1}$$

Thus, the transmission time spent (T_G) corresponds to RTT / 2. Through the results of this experiment, it was possible to obtain the data transmission average time from the biomedical devices to the mobile phone via Bluetooth.

The Fig 14 shows the RTT time spent on all 100 packets. With the RTT time, the T_G time can be calculated and it is shown on Table 1.

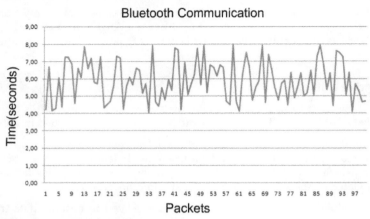

Fig. 14. Time spent on the Bluetooth transmission.

Round trip (RTT) average time	On way trip (T_G) average time
5,91 seconds	2,95 seconds

Table 1. Transmissions average time.

5.2 Cellular local processing

The processing time on the phone is the time taken to compare the current data received from the patient with data patterns previously registered on the device and detect whether or not there is abnormality in the received data.

As mention before, the system has to be previously configured with the patient patterns, as the data references can vary a lot among people.

The Fig 15 shows the time spent for local processing from the 100 packets tested, and the average time.

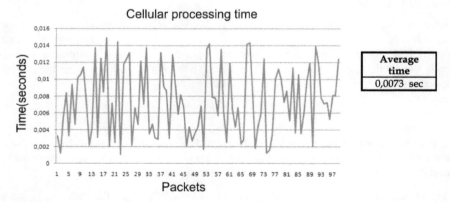

Fig. 15. Time spent on cellular local time processing.

5.3 GPRS transmission time

The GPRS transmission time is the time calculated from the data transmission from the cell until the arrival of the web server. The Fig 16 shows the time and average time spent on the transmission respectively.

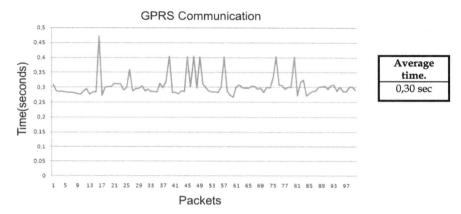

Fig. 16. GPRS transmission time.

5.4 Total transmission time

The total transmission time is summing the three averages presenting in

Table 2. Fig 17 shows the total time obtained along the 100 transmissions. Table 3 shows the average time and the standard deviation of the total time. The Bluetooth transmission is slower also because the synchronization time.

Technology	Time (seconds)
Bluetooth (Monitor to cellular)	2.95
Cellular local processing	0.0073
GPRS (cellular to server)	0.30

Table 2. Average time in the three communication steps.

Times	Time (seconds)
Total average time	3.26
Minimum time	2.32
Maximum time	4.28
Standard deviation	0.57

Table 3. Obtained Results.

The total average time of 3.26s validates the hypothesis that the total transmission time does not compromise the patient's live. This can be confirmed with the standard deviation time which is much lower than the average time. Even the highest time obtained still would not

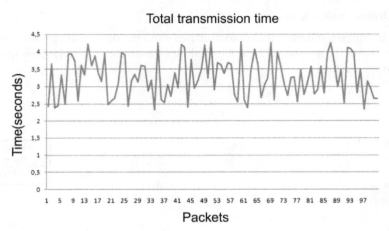

Fig. 17. Total transmission time.

compromise the patient's life. As without the AngelCare, the patient or the family would have to pick up the phone and call an ambulance, resulting in a time higher than 4.28 seconds.

5.5 Angel care advantages and disadvantages

Table 6 shows some advantages and disadvantages of the technology presented. It is important to note that some disadvantages do not come from the technology but from the homecare system itself. There are some points that can vary from each country, especially if we can compare 3rd world countries and 1st world countries. The points presented here are regardless the social class.

Advantages	Disadvantages
Mobility	
Portability	Network dependent
Safeness	Limited choices of medical equipments (homecare disadvantages)
Home environment	Financial (extra cost)
Comfort	
Privacy	

Table 4. AngelCare advantages and disadvantages.

6. Conclusions and future plans

The use of technological innovation in medicine has become extremely important for the scientific advances. This innovation brings the ability to exercise medical surgeries, examinations, consultations in a way never done before and we will all benefit from it. The future of medical technology, judging by their progress accelerated in recent years, leads us to predict that each day there will be new equipment and new diagnostics. The important thing is knowing when to use them and have a clear understanding of its indications, limitations, risks and cost-effective in each particular case.

Ubiquitous computing can be founded among almost all these innovations and allows the junction between the medical needs and the technological power, resulting and new methods and equipments in order to facilitate physician and patient's lives.

This chapter presented a system of remote monitoring for patients who are in homecare and proved to be extremely useful mainly for those who suffer from chronic diseases, or mental disability.

AngelCare is an effective remote monitoring solution for homecare patients. It offers as benefits more mobility, security, comfort and usability in an easy and cheap way and addresses many limitations of current applications

The major contribution of this research was not only the development of a medical system that allows patients monitoring and online access to the data, but it is also the performance analysis of communication and transmission of signals involved. This analysis allowed validating the proposed architecture for homecare patient monitoring. The results obtained in the performance analysis demonstrate the viability and safety of the system since the time between a patient present some abnormality and the arrival of this information in the central server is up to 4.2 seconds, small enough to ensure a fast and efficient care.

Above all, the AngelCare solution can offer a better quality of life to patients and their relatives.

In future plans, AngelCare can be used to monitor all kinds of patients and procedures, as long as the device has a Bluetooth transmission. This wireless and online monitoring has been tested to monitor patient's blood pressure in case of surgery or pos operatory recovering.

7. References

Anatel. Retrieved in: <www.anatel.gov.br>. Acessed in: may, 2011.

Bluetooth. *"Specification of the Bluetooth System."* Version 1.1, Feb. 2001.

Comtech M2M. GPRS tutorial - what is GPRS?. Retrieved from: <http://www.comtechm2m.com/m2m-technology/gprs-tutorial.htm>. Acessed in: february, 2011.

Diane McMichael Gilster Date (2002) . *"Bluetooth end to end"*. ISBN: 0764548875. Published by: Wiley

Figueiredo, C., Nakamura, E. (2003) *"Computação Móvel: Novas Oportunidades e Novos Desafios"*. T&C Amazônia.

Guimarães, R. (2004) *"Bases para uma política nacional de ciência, tecnologia e inovação em saúde."* Ci Saúde Coletiva ; 9(2):375-87. 2.

Hess, C.K., Roman, M., Campbell, R.H., (2002) *"Building Applications for Ubiquitous Computing Environments"*. Proceedings of the Pervasive Computing – First International Conference, p. 16-29.

Java , retrieved in <http://java.sun.com> . Acessed in july 2011.

Kochar, M. S.; Woods, K. D (1990) *"Controle da hipertensão: para enfermeiras e demais profissionais de saúde"*. 2. ed. São Paulo: Andrei. 317p.

Krupinski E. , Nypaver M. , Poropatich R. , Ellis D. , Rihab S., Sapci H. (2002) *"Telemedicine Journal and e-Health"*, Vol. 8, No. 1: 13-34.

Lima, I. (2002) *"Manual do técnico e auxiliar de enfermagem"* - 6ª Edição. Goiânia: AB Editora,, 584p.

Maceratini, Ricardo e Sabattini, Renato M.E. (1994) *"Telemedicina: A Nova Revolução. Revista Informédica."* Volume: 1, Number: 6, Pages: 5-9, January.

Maghsudi M., Hente R., Neumann C., Schachinger U., and Nerlich M. (1999). *"Medical communication from emergency scenes using a notepad computer,"* J. Telemed. Telecare, vol. 5, pp. 249–252.

Mion Jr D, Machado CA, Gomes Mamg et al. (2004) *"IV diretrizes brasileiras de hipertensão arterial"*. Arq Bras Cardiol. 82(Sup IV): 7-22.

Organização Mundial de Saúde (OMS). Retrieved from: <http://www.who.int/en>. Acessed in: december, 2009.

Raffloer K. S. and Wiggens R. A. (1997), *"Video in an ambulance (VIA): wireless multimedia for mobile ambulatory applications,"* in Proc. Amer. Telemed. Assoc. 2nd Annu. Meeting, Atlanta, GA, Apr. 3–6.

Ribeiro, A.G.C.D.; Maitelli, A.L.; Valentim, R.A.M.; Brandão, G.B.; Guerreiro A.M.G; (2010) *"AngelCareAngelCare mobile system: Homecare patient monitoring using Bluetooth and GPRS."* Engineering in Medicine and Biology Society (EMBC), 2010 Annual International Conference of the IEEE. p. 2200 – 2203

Saha, D.;Mukherjee, A. (2003) *"Pervasive computing: A paradigm for the 21st century."* Computer, IEEE Computer Society Press, Los Alamitos, CA, USA, v.36, n.3, p.25-31,2003. ISSN 0018-9162.

Sousa, J. P., Garlan, D. (2002) *"Supporting User Mobility in Ubiquitous Computing Environments"*. Carnegie Mellon University.

Stanford V. (2003) *"Pervasive computing goes the last hundred feet with RFID systems."* IEEE Pervasive Computing; 2: 9-14.

Weiser, M. (1991) *"The Computer for the 21st Century"*. In: Scientific American. Volume: 265, Number: 3, Pages: 94-104, February.

Weiser, M.; Brown, J. (1996). *"Designing Calm Technology."* PowerGrid Journal. Volume: 1, Number: 1, July.

7

Using Brazilian Digital TV to Integrate Health Care Services Embedded in Medical Commercial Devices

Vandermi Silva, Ricardo Erikson Veras De Sena Rosa
and Vicente Ferreira De Lucena Jr.
Federal University of Amazonas, UFAM,
Brazil

1. Introduction

The Digital TV (DTV) System is getting a stimulus within industry and in Brazil that stimulus is based on the belief that this new system will be successful. Several proposals for extending the potential of interactivity, for providing innovative services are available today. In this context, health care is a concept being studied. The health care concept is relative to care about health, in preventing diseases, quality of life and with applications to hospitals, elderly care centres and so on. Integrating health care technology with home devices is a new trend. Thus this chapter shows how the software programmer can integrating devices and sensors with the architecture based in filters presented here.

Our solution is a software platform based on the home gateway, which is in charge of all medical devices interconnecting with the DTV. As proof of the concept, we will build two implementation scenarios. One for measuring heart beat frequency and the other for measuring blood pressure. All the procedures related to the integration are detailed. We believe this work will be useful in this new field, bringing alternative ways for using common devices to provide quality of life to the home user.

The chapter is divided into sections containing foundations, the DTV architecture of health care, construction on a prototype of health care and tests and results, to present the Brazilian standard for digital TV applications and the concepts of health. An overview of the integrated system for medical devices in the architecture section will show an architecture based on filters through all the details and technologies used. In the section on building the prototype we will present how to configure a development environment and how to implement a simple example using the Java programming language and the language Lua. Finally, in the tests and results section illustrations of a system running on a TV will be presented with the Brazilian digital TV standard installed.

1.1 Foundations

The technology improvements in wireless communications and the increasing usage of commercial medical devices to monitor patients have contributed to the development of health care systems targeted to home usage. Indeed, the actual state-of-the-art of these technologies is sufficient to construct highly integrated systems for measuring and collecting patients' data aimed at assisting in diagnoses and prevention of diseases.

In Brazil, according to the Brazilian Institute of Geography and Statistics (IBGE), over 97% of the population living in urban areas have access to television and certainly that percentage should be reflected in the usage of the new digital TV system as soon as it is implemented all over Brazil. Similar studies show that the number of active mobile phones is almost double that of the Brazilian population. This means that almost every family has more than one mobile device available at home.

The IBGE statistics also show that the number people aged 60 years and over in Brazil in 2009 accounted for more than 19 million people. This is 11% of the Brazilian population and the number continues to grow. This study also shows that this population is predicted to reach 30 million over the next 20 years or almost 15% of the population at the end of this period. This leads us to believe that the demand for specialized health services will grow in proportion to the growth of the elderly population, affecting health care in hospitals and nursing homes.

In fact, there is a technological opportunity here. On one hand the market needs applications that automate the processes of monitoring patients remotely to allow for better care quality, reduced queues and costs at the clinics, and on the other hand the Brazilian population has access to new technologies able to construct new equipment and systems that may help solve known problems.

1.1.1 Brazilian DTV

DTV technology is composed of a set of elements comprising signal reception and transmission of the audio and video with digital modulation, a software layer for integrating between the application layer and the hardware, called middleware, and the set of applications. The advance of new algorithms for encoding and decoding audio and video, the transformation of the analogue signal to digital and interactivity via a return channel, allow the viewer a new perspective which will now interact with the DTV system and its programming.

The specification of ISDB-TB standards was based on the Japanese Integrated Services Digital Broadcasting Terrestrial (ISDB-T), following a decision by the Brazilian Digital TV Forum, created by a group led by the National Telecommunications Agency (ANATEL) and the Ministry of Communications. The Brazilian system has been specified with system changes in the compression of audio and video that will now come with encoding H264 and HE-AAC v.2, with speeds up to 30 frames per second.

After defining the standards for all architecture levels of the STB, the Brazilian consortium took charge of the technology to specify the basis of interactivity. In generic architecture of digital TV receivers, the middleware is represented by a software stack that provides an interactive interface for applications to access resources, system services and iDTV. In this regard, the Forum established the Brazilian Ginga as an open standard for the production of interactive programmes and its implementation has been divided into two parts: Ginga-NCL and Ginga-J.

Figure 1 illustrates the Brazilian middleware inserted into the architecture of the STB with ISDB-TB. The subsystem Ginga-J supports Java-based programming, already the Ginga-NCL is focused on the temporal synchronization of media with interactivity. Ginga-NCL follows the model of the Brazilian language NCL (Nested Context Language) that allows the manipulation of media properties to be displayed, event handling, access to information services, etc. In addition to the NCL, the declarative environment of middleware includes another Brazilian programme language called Lua. This subsystem is frequently used and recently Ginga-NCL was recognized as a standard ITU for IPTV.

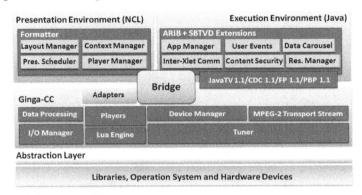

Fig. 1. Ginga middleware architecture.

From the point of view of procedural middleware, Ginga-J is modelled similarly to existing standards, such as JavaTV. The first subsystem specifications included in the software stack of Ginga-J are a set of APIs (Application Programming Interface) for event handling, access to information services, media control, graphical user interface, etc. However, some components of the APIs' platform have been replaced by third-party royalty-free. The specification of the new platform, released in 2009, is based on JavaDTV technology, derived from the Java ME specification for portable consumer devices and modified to suit the peculiarities of the Brazilian digital TV platform.

Currently, the Ginga-J is normalized by the ABNT standard. Two important elements stand out in the Brazilian middleware compared to others in existence: the bridge Ginga-NCL/Ginga-J integration and support communication with multiple devices. The first point refers to a mechanism that allows applications to produce hybrid Ginga-J/Ginga-NCL taking advantage of NCL extensions that allow the application to pass control to other components, that can be written in Java. This enables us to create complete applications that exploit the potential of the platform in its entirety. This mechanism is called common core present in the Ginga, Ginga Common Core or Ginga-CC (see Figure 1): a stack of components that perform functions common to both subsystems.

The second issue is an extension of NCL to enable interaction with other TV devices, such as mobile phones or smartphones. This feature reflects the current trend in digital TV toward connectivity with other devices and can be seen as a potential for the use of other appliances in conjunction with the TV to promote innovative services for users, for example a health care service that integrates mobile systems, medical devices and DTV.

1.1.2 Residential gateway

The Residential Gateway (RG) is a device that interconnects local area network devices with the external environment. The RG focuses management of various services of the residents, providing a single interface to access all devices. In a home network, a given service provider linked through communications technology delivers users functionality implemented by the device, this includes four categories of services that can be distributed on a home network: entertainment (home entertainment), communication (home communications), computer (home computing) and management and monitoring (home monitoring and management). Figure 2 illustrates the role of GR in a home network.

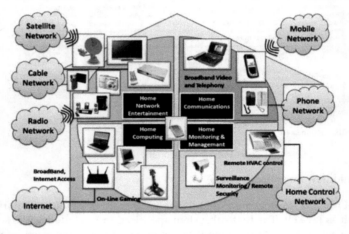

Fig. 2. Network services centralized in the RG. Adapted from O. B. Maia.

To centre on RGfor all types of services, considering the particularities of each, it is necessary to have a software platform that meets the needs of the home environment. Some studies in the literature do an analysis of existing technologies, among which are: Jini, UPnP (Universal Plug and Play) and OSGi (Open Services Gateway Initiative).

To facilitate the integration with medical devices and scenarios for the RG health care is essential. Moreover, as an extension of interactive digital TV, a similar proposal is currently being studied with regard to RG , that being can services be accessed from all devices in the home through DTV.

1.1.3 Medical devices

Currently there are a range of medical devices on the market that can be integrated with systems for the diagnosis and monitoring of chronic diseases. Among these devices are automatic blood pressure meters and pulseoximeters. The combined use of medical devices in a home network for treatment and prevention of disease is already quite common in developed countries like the US and EU countries. In these countries, it is possible to monitor a patient in his own residence. In Brazil, the initiative at the State University of Campinas (Unicamp) which is implementing the concept of a digital city where a backbone will connect all essential services, such as rescue and police, in a short period of time will also be a reality. Some of the most widely used medical devices are shown in Figure 3. There are data collection devices for systolic and diastolic pressure, metering devices of heartbeat and of insulin in the literature able to be integrated with mobile phones or even with small devices, such as a watch.

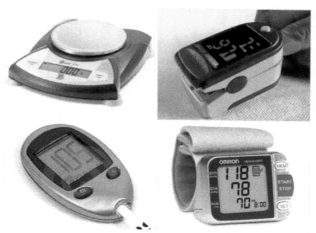

Fig. 3. Example of medical devices.

1.2 DTV Health care architecture

The architectural model of this paper is based on the pipes and filters architecture, which consists of treating the data by applying filters at various levels and transforming the raw data collected from the devices in readable information to the user. Pipes and filters consider the existence of a network through which data flows from one end to another source and the destination data stream undergoes transformations by means of filters. In this work, pipes and filters are unidirectional, leading and treating the data between the source (sensors for medical devices) and destination (RG and DTV).

From the architectural design of the model presented in Figure 4 the system uses two data filters who work in the transformation of the data received from the devices and communication protocols defining a parser that converts the data format to another representation. After the work of these filters, a common document is generated, validated and stored in the database.

The data flow that goes from sensors to the database first passes through a filter of protocols that treat the raw data to then process it into a sub-parser module that generates the document containing the sensor readings. The standard representation generated by the parser is checked by sub-module validator and the result is stored in the database.

From the generation of a data document that can be accessed by all modules of the validator and confirmation as to the origin and formatting of the document, the second filter data using the module action queries the document to verify that the values in pressure and heart rate are consistent with those stipulated by the health professional.

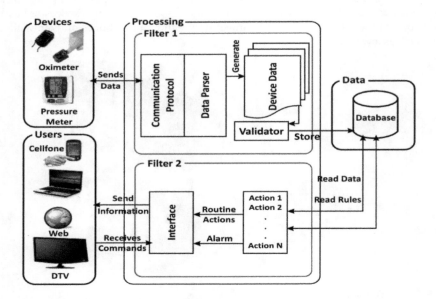

Fig. 4. Proposed architecture based in filters.

Through an interface with the devices that display data to the user, such as phones, computers connected to the Web and STB platforms with standard Brazilian DTV, the messaging subsystem, through action routines, performs the task of sending SMS messages (or prompts for TVDi).

The action module needs to check a table of rules for sending messages to the cell and the DTV. Therefore, based on the literature found in the area of health, a document containing such rules should be developed and stored in the database. Two examples of such data can be seen in Tables 1 and 2, respectively, showing the maximum range of the expected heart rate for an individual exercise and classification of blood pressure in adults over 18 years.

To illustrate the process, assume a scenario of monitoring the physical activity of a person on a treadmill. The user while performing the activity with a medical device (heart rate meter) attached generates raw data that are passed to the controller (a filter in Figure 4), enabling the execution of the components of the protocol level, which will address the data and store the useful information in the database. Then, obeying the rule base previously stored, the system (two components of the filter in Figure 4) checks the new data, sending the inferences made from the base of rules applied to the corresponding information. The result could be a message that appears on the TVDi, such as: "slow down the activity you are doing is too much physical effort."

The main challenges to implementing the solution are the integration of conventional medical devices with DTV, the synchronization between the devices when accessing the database and the implementation of common rules for the preparation of messages to be

Age	Max Freq.	Ideal Freq. 75%	Target zone between 70% and 80%
20	200	150	140 and 170
25	195	146	137 and 166
30	190	142	133 and 162
35	185	139	130 and 157
40	180	135	126 and 153
45	175	131	123 and 149
50	170	127	119 and 145
60	160	120	112 and 136
65	155	116	109 and 132
70	150	116	105 and 128

Table 1. Maximum heart rate range. [29]

Systolic	Diastolic	Category
greater than 130	less than 85	Normal
130-139	85-89	Normal Height
140-159	90-99	Mild hypertension (Stage 1)
160-179	100-119	Moderate hypertension (Stage 2)
180-209	110-119	Severe hypertension (Stage 3)
equal to the greater 210	equal to the greater 210	Hypertension very severe (Stage 4)

Table 2. Classification of blood pressure in adults aged less than 18 years. [28]

posted on the display devices. This is partly because there is no standardization of data sent by the devices, because each manufacturer uses its own standards and protocols for generation and transmission of sensor data.

1.2.1 Scenarios for architecture implementation

One scenario that can be used for implementation is the use of a mobile phone to send alert messages to users of a health care system. Thus, a module can send messages using a messaging library that can be integrated into the architecture of GR as a return channel of the application. In this study we used an API written in Java that can be found at http://smslib.org/. In the section on construction of the prototype we will demonstrate how to use the API.

The architecture scenario of the module Short Message System (SMS) is illustrated in Figure 5 and runs on the layer of JVM (Java Virtual Machine) installed on GR. Thus, a text message can be triggered for devices registered with the GR, using the infrastructure network of Global System for Mobile Communications (GSM) and its communication protocols.

In this scenario presented in Figure 5, two mobile devices must be present: a cell associated with the GR and another target, whose number is stored in the database. If any medical device presents a reading in a range of risk, considering the rules of the tables on module action, the GR uses a cellular network as an output for sending data over the Internet. The

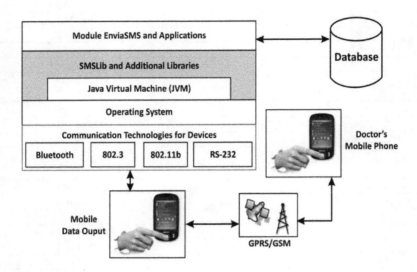

Fig. 5. Module for sending SMS messages.

SMSLib enable communication through this module EnviaSMS. Once connected to the cell output, the GR sends the alert message (blood pressure or heart rate) for the device registered in the database, which can be the phone of the doctor or person responsible for the monitored patient.

For the presentation of messages on a mobile device, Micro-edition Java (J2ME) can be used, which has a Java virtual machine for devices with low processing power (KVM). From the application layer there is access to layers of Profile and Mobile Information Device Profile (MIDP) that allow direct access to the layer Connected Limited Device Configuration (CLDC), responsible for device configurations accessible to the Kilobyte Virtual Machine (KVM), a custom Java virtual machine to the limitations of devices with low processing power.

The application layer is limited to the use of CLDC with MIDP, to reduce the cost of memory and processing power, enabling low-cost handsets to be used in the implementation of the prototypes. Figure 6 illustrates the modules that make up the JME platform, inserted into the overall system architecture.

Finally, a presentation module of the data in DTV can be built using the architecture shown in Figure 7. Within this module is an interface to an application using DTV Brazilian Ginga middleware technologies. For the two sub-specifications of middleware, applications were built corresponding: to the Java part, considering also the unavailability of an open platform 100% compatible with the Ginga-J, we adopted a subset of the MHP middleware API. For the environment we created a declarative interface for data visualization in NCLua. The data is accessed via APIs specific to each platform.

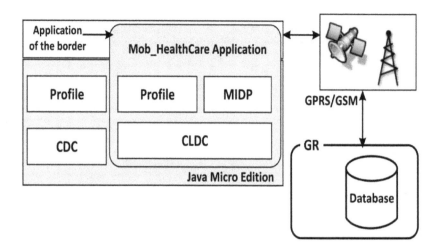

Fig. 6. Module of the mobile device architecture J2ME.

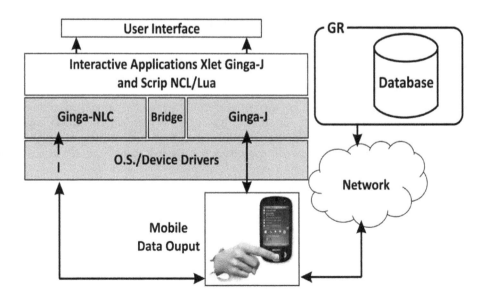

Fig. 7. Architecture for DTV module.

The alert module receives the data via the network through the reading of the GR database and then displays that data on the screen of the DTV. On submission of alerts, the GR first queries the database to see if it is a new alert, then sends it to the DTV module that displays it on the screen. The user, through the remote control, can access information on devices and decide to perform a procedure on the patient, depending on what is recommended by the system.

1.3 Building your health care software prototype

To assemble the test environment of the proposed model we incorporated technologies on the market for each of the components of the modules of Figures 5, 6 and 7. Among the solutions used were the XBee as a means of communication between the GR and the oximeter, GSM networks for the transmission of information relating to medical devices and XML to build a model for the standardization of information.

The hardware of the GR is designed on the x86 architecture, comprising a dual-core Atom processor, motherboard model A945GC with gigabit Ethernet interfaces, sound, video, 1GB of RAM and at least 8GB for storage, where we set up the System Linux operating system and related applications.

1.3.1 Installing and configuring the gateway

The operating system used at the time this chapter was written was the Linux Ubuntu 10.10, but new versions of Linux based on Debian will also work. To install Ubuntu 10.10 it is necessary to start the gateway computer via CD and run the installation from it. A tutorial that explains step by step installation of Ubuntu can be found at the link https: //help.ubuntu.com/10.10/installation-guide/. After installing the operating system, you must install the Java development tools, it is enough to open the terminal command as the Linux root user and run the command add-apt-repository "deb http://archive. canonical.com/ Lucidpartner " and then apt-get install sun-java6-jre sun-java6-jdk.

After the configuration of Java, you must install the RXTXLinux API that will allow access to data from the serial port device connected to the gateway. Simply download the API directly from wiki http://rtx.qbang.org/wiki. To Linux systems, you can insert the lib RXTcomm.jar in the folder /jre/lib/ext and insert the librxtxSerial.so too. Make sure the user is in group lock or uucp so lockfiles work.

1.3.2 Application configurations

Before starting the development it is ideal to set up a directory structure similar to that shown in Figure 8, to separate the data collected from sensors and devices, and other parts of the implementation.

The folder includes the gateway application app folder in which should be installed the data collector and folder date, responsible for storing data generated in the XML file. To generate the XML API you can use any Java-compatible, however in the example shown we used the API JDOM parser which was already integrated and easy to use.

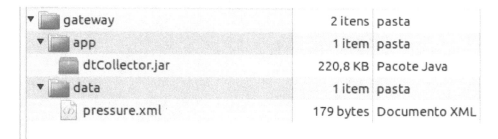

▼ 📁 gateway	2 itens	pasta
▼ 📁 app	1 item	pasta
📁 dtCollector.jar	220,8 KB	Pacote Java
▼ 📁 data	1 item	pasta
📄 pressure.xml	179 bytes	Documento XML

Fig. 8. Folder structure of the application.

1.3.3 Encoding an example using a pressure meter

We will now present an example coding of data collection of a blood pressure meter. For this example we used the measuring device shown in Figure 3 that can be easily found on the market. This device was connected to the gateway via a USB cable. Then the software collector runs, reads the USB port, collects data and stores them in an XML file. An example of the XML file stored is shown in Figure 9, where we can see the storage of data from the pressure meter already treated and ready to be presented in DTV.

```
*pressure.xml ✖
<?xml version="1.0" encoding="UTF-8"?>
<pressure>
        <patient>
                <name>John</name>
                <systolic>120</systolic>
                <diastolic>80</diastolic>
        </patient>
</pressure>
```

Fig. 9. XML data collecting by application.

To generate the XML file shown, it is necessary to codify the first reading from the USB port, so that a class written in Java was developed. This class has methods for reading the specific USB port, decoding of bytes received on the port, the transformation of information using substrings and finally creating the data file into XML using JDOM API. Parts of the source code showing the constructed methods are presented in Figure 10 and then its operation is explained.

The SerialEvent method shown in Figure 10 checks the bytes being passed into the USB port, synchronizes with the device using a second, and checks if the buffer has received some information. If you have an error while reading an exception is thrown and the method aborts execution. This method treats the events in serial or USB port connected on the device and uses the rxtx API for this.

```
// Event manager for serial/USB port
      public void serialEvent(SerialPortEvent ev) {

            switch (ev.getEventType()) {
            case SerialPortEvent.BI:
            case SerialPortEvent.OE:
            case SerialPortEvent.FE:
            case SerialPortEvent.PE:
            case SerialPortEvent.CD:
            case SerialPortEvent.CTS:
            case SerialPortEvent.DSR:
            case SerialPortEvent.RI:
            case SerialPortEvent.OUTPUT_BUFFER_EMPTY:
                  break;|
            case SerialPortEvent.DATA_AVAILABLE:
                  byte[] bufferLeitura = new byte[6];
                  try {
                        Thread.sleep(1000); //sincronize with device 1 second
                        while (inputStream.available() > 0) {
                              nodeBytes = inputStream.read(bufferLeitura);
                        }

                        if (bufferLeitura.length == 0) {
                              System.out.println("nothing read!");
                        } else if (bufferLeitura.length == 1) {
                              System.out.println("a byte was reading!");
                        } else {
                              getDados(bufferLeitura);
                        }
                  } catch (Exception e) {
                        System.out.println("[ ERROR ] Error during reading: " + e);
                  }
                  break;
            }
      }
```

Fig. 10. Event Manager for serial/USB ports.

Another part of the source of importance and worth noting is the method getDados. This method works with substrings to separate the information and extract only the necessary data. This is because the pressure measuring device sends a set of bits via serial port that include heart rate, systolic pressure, diastolic pressure and time of data collection. This example was not required to collect all information and thus we concentrated our efforts on separating only the systolic and diastolic blood pressure to generate the document data.

Figure 11 shows part of the method getDados and the logic as separate substrings. First, the method converts the information received in bytes, for strings, then counts the characters and stores them into substrings. Then it finds the position of the token and appends the information to finally send to the method that generates the data file. This process is repeated until all data is collected and treated. In the next step, the data file in XML format is created in the folder "data" of the gateway, which can be accessed via DTV using a wireless network connection. Part of the source code that generates the XML file is shown in Figure 12.

Looking at the source code in Figure 12, it is clear that data handled are passed as parameters to be inserted in the XML file using the method FileWriter. The JDOM API methods create the tags in accordance with the custom configuration for the client. For example, if the client wants to enter the patient's name, it is passed as a parameter to the application that generates the tag name.

```
public String getDados(byte[] b) throws Exception {
        //using substring for process the data
        String r1 = "";
        String r2 = "";
        String r3 = "";
        String r4 = "";
        String r5 = "";
        String r6 = "";
        @SuppressWarnings("unused")
        String conc1 = "";
        String conc2 = "";
        String[] resfinal = new String[3];
        String result = "";
        String result2 = "";

        // dividing the values of the read
        for (int i = 0; i < b.length; i++) {
                result += Integer.toString((b[i] & 0xff) + 0x100, 16).substring(1);
                result2 += Integer.parseInt(Integer.toString((b[i] & 0xff) + 0x100,
                                16).substring(1), 16);

                //verify size 12 characters
                if (result2.length() == 12) {

                        r1 = result2.substring(0, 2);
                        r2 = result2.substring(2, 4);
                        r3 = result2.substring(4, 6);
                        r4 = result2.substring(6, 8);
                        r5 = result2.substring(8, 10);
                        r6 = result2.substring(10, 12);

                //token position
                if ((Integer.parseInt(r1) == 13)
                                && (Integer.parseInt(r2) == 25)) {
                        conc1 = r3.substring(0, 1);
                        conc2 = r3.substring(1, 2);
                        resfinal[0] = (conc2 + r4);
                        resfinal[1] = r5;
                        resfinal[2] = r6;
                        getValidations(resfinal);
                }|
```

Fig. 11. Part of the source code of the method getDados.

```
//XML file generate for DTV
        public Element getXMLPressure(String nome, String sist, String dist)
                        throws Exception {

                //using JDOM API
                Element pressure = new Element("pressure");
                Document doc_pressure = new Document(pressure);

                Element pacient = criarElementXml(nome, sist, dist);
                pressure.addContent(pacient);

                XMLOutputter xout = new XMLOutputter();
                try {

                        FileWriter arquivo_alerta = new FileWriter(new File(FILE_PATH));

                        xout.output(doc_pressure, arquivo_alerta);

                } catch (IOException e) {
                        e.printStackTrace();
                }

                return pacient;

        }
```

Fig. 12. getXMLPressure method.

1.4 Results presented at the DTV

To display the monitoring data was used in a DTV STBs, with a Brazilian middleware Ginga-NCL that supports interactive applications that can run an external storage device or transmitted directly to the STB via broadcast by the broadcaster.

For the data presentation using the specification in DTV Ginga-NCL there were certain changes in the architecture, because the programming structure of NCL/Lua and JavaTV differs from the API. Currently in Brazil, most STBs compatible with the national standard have not yet run code written in Java. However, some companies have their own versions of middleware that enable execution of applications written in NCL and Lua. According to the programming model to the Ginga-NCL, an application to access the XML data from GR by extending the functionality of the application through the NCL script Lua has been developed.

In NCL are defined items responsible for the presentation of media (images, videos, text) and user interaction with the remote control. Through a link element control of the application for a Lua script can pass which performs a specific function and returns control to the NCL.

In this case, with regard to the health care application system, the Lua script is responsible for establishing a TCP / IP with GR, retrieving and processing the data in XML, and then formatting them for display on screen TVDi.

Figures 13 illustrates, respectively, a warning to the interface pressure measurement and presentation of data collected from GR, after you connect medical devices to the system. The interface was built in NCL / Moon in a real STB.

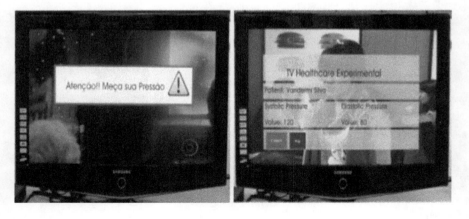

Fig. 13. Data presented at the DTV.

Part of the source code responsible for reading the XML and display of the DTV is shown in Figure 14.

```lua
--[[Class control
        responsable by read XML
        XML
--]]
parserXML = {

loadFile = function( nome_arquivo )
    local arquivo = io.open (nome_arquivo) , "r"        -- open file
    local texto = ""                                    -- Criate array
    for linha in arquivo:lines() do
        if linha:len() > 0 then
            texto = texto .. linha .. '\n'

        end
    end
    return texto
end,

parseargs = function(s)
  local arg = {}
  string.gsub(s, "(%w+)=([\"'])(.-)%2", function (w, _, a)
    arg[w] = a
  end)
  return arg
end,
```

Fig. 14. Source code in Lua.

```xml
<?xml version="1.0" encoding="ISO-8859-1"?>
<ncl id="chat_tela" xmlns="http://www.ncl.org.br/NCL3.0/EDTVProfile">
        <head>
                <regionBase>
                        <region id="rgVideoFullscreen" zIndex="1"/>
                        <region id="rgLua" width="100%" height="100%" right="0" top="0" zIndex="10" />
                </regionBase>

                <descriptorBase>
                        <descriptor id="dVideoFullscreen"  region="rgVideoFullscreen"/>
                        <descriptor id="dLua" region="rgLua" focusIndex="1" />
                </descriptorBase>
        </head>

        <body>
                <!--port id="pVideoAbertura" component="videoAbertura"/-->
                <port id="pLua" component="lua" />

                <media id="lua" src="main.lua" descriptor="dLua" />
                <media id="videoAbertura" src="sbtvd-ts://0" descriptor="dVideoFullscreen" />
                <!--media id="videoAbertura" src="img/background.jpg" descriptor="dVideoFullscreen" /-->
        </body>
</ncl>
```

Fig. 15. Source code in NCL.

The script uses a Lua function that captures the XML file stored on the server through the LAN and shares your information to further the application developed in NCL graphically presented in DTV. This is possible because the Ginga-NCL enables integration between Lua and NCL, which allows working static and dynamic content on DTV.

We hope this chapter serves as a first step to assist readers who want to better understand how technologies can be integrated to develop applications for day to day users. The work is hard, but certainly rewarding.

2. References

[1] IBGE. Instituto Brasileiro de Geografia e Estatística. "Pesquisa Nacional por Amostragem de Domicílios".
    http://www.ibge.gov.br. Acessado em 01/06/2011.
[2] CNDH. Coordenação Nacional de Hipertensão e Diabetes.
    http://dab.saude.gov.br/cnhd. Acessado em 01/06/2011
[3] SBTVD. Fórum Brasileiro de TV Digital.
    http://www.forumsbtvd.org.br/. Acessado em: 01/06/2011.
[4] S. Morris, A. Smith-Chaigneau. Interactive TV Standards A Guide to MHP, OCAP and Java TV. Burlington, MA, USA: Elsevier, 608p, 2005.
[5] ABNT. Associação Brasileira de Normas Técnicas. "NBR 15606-2:2007. Televisão Digital Terrestre – Codificação de dados e Especificações de Transmissão para Radiodifusão Digital – Parte 2: Ginga-NCL para Receptores Fixos e Móveis – Linguagem de aplicação XML para codificação de aplicações".
[6] L. F. G. Soares, M. F. Moreno, C. S. Neto. "Ginga-NCL: Declarative Middleware for Multimedia IPTV Services". IEEE. Communications Magazine, Vol. 48, No. 6, p. 74-81, 2010.
[7] R. Ierusalimschy Programming in Lua. Rio de Janeiro: Editora da Pontifícia Universidade Católica do Rio de Janeiro (PUC-RIO), 327p, 2006.
[8] M. F. Moreno, C. E. C. F. Batista, L. F. G. Soares. "NCL and ITU-T's Standardization Effort on Multimedia Application Frameworks for IPTV". Brazilian Symposium on Multimedia and Web, Vol. 1, No. 1, p. 1-6, 2010.
[9] M. Legally, J. Pätzold. "New TV Standard for Digital TV in Brazil".
    http://download.java.net/mobileembedded/developerdays/2009/TS-5-v2.pdf. Acessado em 01/06/2011.
[10] M. F. Moreno, L. F. G. Soares. "Resilient Hypermedia Presentations". IEEE Workshop on Software Aging and Rejuvenation (WoSAR), Vol. 1, No. 1, p. 1-6, 2011.
[11] G. L. de Souza Filho, L. E. C. Leite, C. E. Batista. "Ginga-J: The procedural middleware for the Brazilian digital TV system". Journal of the Brazilian Computer Society, Vol. 13, No. 1, p. 47-56, 2007.
[12] ABNT. Associação Brasileira de Normas Técnicas. ABNT NBR 15606-4. Part 4: Ginga-J – The Environment for the Execution of Procedural Applications.

[13] L. F. G. Soares, R. M. Costa, M. F. Moreno. "Multiple exhibition Devices in DTV systems". *MM'09 Proceedings of the 17th ACM International Conference on Multimedia*, Vol. 1, No. 1, p. 281-290, 2009.

[14] O. B. Maia, N. S. Viana, V. F. de Lucena Jr. "Using the iDTV as a Center of a Ubiquitous Computing Environment". *InTech Open Publisher Access*, Vol. 1, No. 1, p. 225-248, 2011.

[15] N. S. Viana; V. F. de Lucena Jr., "iDTV Home Gateway Convergence: an Open Software Model Integrating the Ginga Middleware and the OSGi Framework". *Multimedia Systems*, Vol.16, No.5, p. 1-15, 2010.

[16] S. Dixit, R. Prasad. "Technologies for Home Networking". New York: John Wiley & Sons, 218p, 2008.

[17] V. F. de Lucena Jr., J. E. C. Filho, N. S. Viana, O. B. Maia. "A Home Automation Proposal Built on the Ginga Digital TV Middleware and the OSGi Framework". *IEEE Transactions on Consumer Electronics*, Vol. 55, No. 3, p. 1254-1262, 2009.

[18] W. –W Lin, Yu-Hsiang-Sheng. "Using OSGi, UPnP and Zigbee to Provide a Wireless Ubiquitous Home Healthcare Environment". *IEEE Computer Society*, Vol. 1, No. 1, p. 268-272, 2008.

[19] R. C. Augusto, J. Carlos, S. Daniel. "Ambient Intelligence — The Next Step for Artificial Intelligence". *IEEE Intelligent Systems*, Vol. 23, No. 2, p. 15–18, 2008. ISSN 1541-1672.

[20] J. Corchado, J. Bajo, J. Abraham. "Healthcare Delivery IN Geriatric Residences". *IEEE Intelligent Systems*, Vol. 23, No. 2, p. 19-25, 2008.

[21] M. Valero, L. Vadillo. "An Implementation Framework for Smart Home Telecare Services". *Future Generation Communication and Networking (FCGN)*, Vol. 2, No. 1, p. 60–65, 2007.

[22] PROTÉGÉ. Overview. http://protege.stanford.edu/overview/. Acessado em 01/06/2011.

[23] D. S. G. Pekhteryev, H. Z. Sahinoglu, C. Challa. "Cam N. Real-Time and Secure Wireless Health Monitoring". Int. J. Telemedicine Appl. Computer, Vol. 1, No. 1, p. 1-10, 2008.

[24] V. Becker, L. F. Soares. "Viva Mais Alimentação Saudável". http://clube.ncl.org.br/node/29. Acessado em 01/06/2011.

[25] V. Becker, L. F. Soares. "Viva Mais Peso Ideal". http://clube.ncl.org.br/node/15. Acessado em 01/06/2011.

[26] Portal do Software Público Brasileiro. Governo Federal. http://www.softwarepublico.gov.br/. Acessado em 01/06/2011.

[27] A. Mendes. Arquitetura de Software: Desenvolvimento Orientado para a Arquitetura. Rio de Janeiro, RJ, Brasil: Campus, 212p, 2002.

[28] F. de C. Branco, J. M. Viana, J. R. P. Lima. "Freqüência Cardíaca na Prescrição de Treinamento de Corredores de Fundo". *R. Bras. Ci. e Mov.*, Vol. 12, No. 2, p. 75-79, 2004.

[29] Chobanian, A. V. et al. Seventh report of the joint national committee on prevention, detection, evaluation, and treatment of high blood pressure. the American Heart Association, v. 1, n. 1, p. 1221–1222, December 2003.

Permissions

The contributors of this book come from diverse backgrounds, making this book a truly international effort. This book will bring forth new frontiers with its revolutionizing research information and detailed analysis of the nascent developments around the world.

We would like to thank Ranjit Sahu and Shaul Mordechai, for lending their expertise to make the book truly unique. They have played a crucial role in the development of this book. Without their invaluable contribution this book wouldn't have been possible. They have made vital efforts to compile up to date information on the varied aspects of this subject to make this book a valuable addition to the collection of many professionals and students.

This book was conceptualized with the vision of imparting up-to-date information and advanced data in this field. To ensure the same, a matchless editorial board was set up. Every individual on the board went through rigorous rounds of assessment to prove their worth. After which they invested a large part of their time researching and compiling the most relevant data for our readers. Conferences and sessions were held from time to time between the editorial board and the contributing authors to present the data in the most comprehensible form. The editorial team has worked tirelessly to provide valuable and valid information to help people across the globe.

Every chapter published in this book has been scrutinized by our experts. Their significance has been extensively debated. The topics covered herein carry significant findings which will fuel the growth of the discipline. They may even be implemented as practical applications or may be referred to as a beginning point for another development. Chapters in this book were first published by InTech; hereby published with permission under the Creative Commons Attribution License or equivalent.

The editorial board has been involved in producing this book since its inception. They have spent rigorous hours researching and exploring the diverse topics which have resulted in the successful publishing of this book. They have passed on their knowledge of decades through this book. To expedite this challenging task, the publisher supported the team at every step. A small team of assistant editors was also appointed to further simplify the editing procedure and attain best results for the readers.

Our editorial team has been hand-picked from every corner of the world. Their multi-ethnicity adds dynamic inputs to the discussions which result in innovative outcomes. These outcomes are then further discussed with the researchers and contributors who give their valuable feedback and opinion regarding the same. The feedback is then collaborated with the researches and they are edited in a comprehensive manner to aid the understanding of the subject.

Apart from the editorial board, the designing team has also invested a significant amount of their time in understanding the subject and creating the most relevant covers. They scrutinized every image to scout for the most suitable representation of the subject and create an appropriate cover for the book.

The publishing team has been involved in this book since its early stages. They were actively engaged in every process, be it collecting the data, connecting with the contributors or procuring relevant information. The team has been an ardent support to the editorial, designing and production team. Their endless efforts to recruit the best for this project, has resulted in the accomplishment of this book. They are a veteran in the field of academics and their pool of knowledge is as vast as their experience in printing. Their expertise and guidance has proved useful at every step. Their uncompromising quality standards have made this book an exceptional effort. Their encouragement from time to time has been an inspiration for everyone.

The publisher and the editorial board hope that this book will prove to be a valuable piece of knowledge for researchers, students, practitioners and scholars across the globe.

List of Contributors

Asmaa Hatem Rashid and Norizan Binti Mohd Yasin
Department of Information Science, Faculty of Computer Science and IT, University of Malaya, Kuala Lampur, Malaysia

Luís Velez Lapão
Instituto de Higiene e Medicina Tropical, Universidade Nova de Lisboa, CINTESIS: Center for Research in Health Technologies and Information Systems, Universidade do Porto, Portugal

Malgorzata Plechawska-Wojcik
Lublin University of Technology, Poland

Tayeb Merabti, Julien Grosjean and Stefan J. Darmoni
CISMeF, Rouen University Hospital, Normandy & TIBS, LITIS EA 4108, Institute of Biomedical Research, Rouen, France

Lina F. Soualmia
CISMeF, Rouen University Hospital, Normandy & TIBS, LITIS EA 4108, Institute of Biomedical Research, Rouen, France
LIM & Bio EA 3969, Paris XIII University, Sorbonne Paris Cité, Bobigny, France

Michel Joubert
LERTIM EA 3283, Faculty of Medicine, Marseilles, France

Hsueh-Chun Lin
Department of Health Risk Management, School of Public Health, China Medical University, Taichung, Taiwan

Anna G. C. D. Ribeiro, André L. Maitelli, Ricardo A. M. Valentim and Ana M. G. Guerreiro
Laboratory of Hospital Automation and Bioengineering, Federal University of Rio Grande do Norte, Brazil

Cicília Raquel Maia Leite
State University of Rio Grande do Norte, Brazil

Vandermi Silva, Ricardo Erikson Veras De Sena Rosa and Vicente Ferreira De Lucena Jr.
Federal University of Amazonas, UFAM, Brazil